Paediatric Revision

Paediatric Revision

Kwei C. Chin MB ChB (Glasgow) MRCP (UK) DCH
Consultant Paediatrician
St Peter's Hospital, Chertsey, Surrey

Formerly Lecturer in Paediatrics and Child Health
University of Birmingham,
East Birmingham Hospital,
Birmingham

Michael J. Tarlow MB Bs MSc FRCP (London)
Senior Lecturer in Paediatrics and Child Health,
University of Birmingham,
East Birmingham Hospital,
Birmingham

Churchill Livingstone 🏛
LONDON EDINBURGH MELBOURNE AND NEW YORK 1989

CHURCHILL LIVINGSTONE
Medical Division of Longman Group UK Limited

Distributed in the United States of America by
Churchill Livingstone Inc., 1560 Broadway, New
York, N.Y. 10036, and by associated companies,
branches and representatives throughout the
world.

First published 1989

ISBN 0-443-03274-2

British Library Cataloguing in Publication Data
Chin, Kwei C.
    Paediatric revision.
    1. Paediatrics — Questions & answers
    I. Title   II. Tarlow, Michael J.
    618.92'00076

Library of Congress Cataloging in Publication Data
Chin, Kwei C.
    Paediatric revision.
    1. Pediatrics — Examinations, questions, etc.
I. Tarlow, Michael J.   II. Title.   [DNLM: 1. Pediatrics
examination questions. WS 18 C539p]
RJ48.2.C47   1989   618.92'00076   88-20382

Produced by Longman Singapore Publishers (Pte) Ltd.
Printed in Singapore

Foreword

Failing an examination because of lack of medical knowledge or clinical competence is bad enough (and also expensive), but failing an examination because of lack of knowledge about how that examination is constructed and how the marks are awarded is even worse. Sadly, many candidates in examinations do not make the most of their knowledge and skills and do not provide answers or perform in the ways that score most marks, and of which they are capable.

Examiners, for their part, try to conduct examinations as fairly as possible and seek to discriminate correctly between the good candidate and the bad. I doubt if there are any medical examinations in Britain over which more detailed care is taken in the construction of questions, arrangements for the clinical examination, and in the assessment of questions, and of examiners, as the MRCP examination. Yet all too often candidates seem to fail because of a lack of awareness of how to answer questions in the best way and how to utilise fully their clinical skills. There is no secret about how the DCH and the MRCP examinations are constructed or how marks are awarded, yet candidates often behave as if they are unaware of the basic information given in the first section of this book.

Examiners, as well as candidates, will welcome the dissemination of this information and also the carefully prepared sections relating to case histories, data interpretation, projected material and multiple choice questions.

For any candidate this book is useful preparation for a paediatric examination; it provides a way of learning as well as a way of revising. The best use comes from tackling the book seriously (and not cheating by looking at the answers first), and forcing oneself to consider the question carefully, then committing oneself firmly to an answer before looking up the correct answer. Thus casual reading gives way to efficient reading and programmed learning.

Dr Chin and Dr Tarlow are experienced teachers who have met more than their fair share of candidates working for our examinations in paediatrics. They know the sort of book those candidates need, and they have provided it.

1989   Roy Meadow

Introduction

This book has developed out of the postgraduate courses in paediatrics that were established at East Birmingham Hospital in the mid-1970s and have continued since. The courses are designed as part of a revision course in paediatrics and are suitable for those individuals who are planning to take a higher examination in the subject.

Although the types of question asked reflect those of the British MRCP and DCH examinations, it is hoped that those undergoing paediatric training in other countries will also find the book helpful and informative. We would suggest it be used as an adjunct to structured revision, in addition to the many outstanding tests that already exist in general and specialty paediatrics.

The questions are intended to concentrate on the relevant and important rather than the trivial or the specious; we have tried to stress the importance of precision both in the use and understanding of words, and in tightly delineating an answer.

Mistakes have undoubtedly been made, both in emphasis and in fact, despite careful checking and rechecking of the whole book. Please write to us correcting our mistakes so that they do not get carried through into possible future editions.

Birmingham, 1989   K.C.C.
M.J.T.

Acknowledgements

We would like to thank all our colleagues who have contributed to the East Birmingham Teaching Courses over the years and thus directly or indirectly to this book. We would particularly name Doctors Geoff Durbin, Andrea Mayne, Jeff Bissenden, Jeremy Allgrove and Geoff Lawson, for their unstinting assistance; Megan Wood and Marianne Joseph for their administrative and organisational help, and Elaine Kindred and Suzanne Harrison for typing the manuscripts. Finally we owe a debt of gratitude to all the doctors who have come on our courses and have helped us improve the precision and accuracy of the questions.

Finally, our thanks to Fisons plc and Glaxo Laboratories Ltd whose generous sponsorship enabled us to use colour in the Projected material section.

Kwei Chin
Michael Tarlow

Contents

I Introduction

INTRODUCTION

Since December 1972, the three Royal Colleges of Physicians (London, Edinburgh and Glasgow) have been holding a common Part 2 examination. It is held simultaneously by the three Colleges. From 1977, paediatricians in training have had their own Part 2 examination in paediatrics. However, successful candidates in paediatrics or general medicine will be awarded the MRCP (UK) diploma without any differentiation between the specialities. The examination consists of the written section, clinicals and oral examination. Only those candidates who have passed the written paper are certain to proceed to the clinical examination. Candidates who have marginally failed may also be invited to attend the clinicals. Aim not to be in this group!

THE WRITTEN EXAMINATION

This section consists of three parts:

1. The case histories.
2. Data interpretation.
3. Projected material.

Each part of the written examination is designed to test certain aspects of the candidates' abilities (see details under each part). The examination is also designed to require minimal writing but lots of thought.

Note: Normal case histories, data and slides are likely to be included. Answers like 'normal' or 'no treatment required' or 'reassure parents' are all that may be required.

General approach

- Read each question very carefully. This cannot be over-emphasized.
- Answers should be concise, specific and complete. Do not write sentences. Do not give explanations for your answers. Do not give vague answers.
- If the question asks for one diagnosis or two investigations, give the *required* number of answers. Extra answers do not attract extra marks. Furthermore, only the *first* answer is accepted even if the second answer is better.
- Answer all the questions. If in difficulty, move on to the next but leave time to come back to the difficult ones.
- When faced with a difficult question, do not panic! Refer back to the history and/or data. Try to list down all the important positive and negative features. Ask yourself the significance of each feature. A systematic approach is more likely to be fruitful. Remember that your best answer must be based only on whatever information that is given in the question.
- Avoid using abbreviations.
- Lastly, write legibly.

The marking system

The marking of the written examination is very fair. Each college takes it in turn to mark different parts of the examination. Furthermore, to the examiners the candidates are anonymous and are identified by examination numbers only.

- There is a *scaled marking system* for each question. As decided by the Examination Board, the best answer(s) carries the top mark and the 'not-so-good' answer gets less or no marks (e.g. +4 for best answer to 0 mark).
- In the three sections each question may carry a different maximum mark.
- But all three parts of the written examination carry the *same* maximum marks.
- The *pass* mark is said to be the average of the three papers.
- If the first part of the answer is completely wrong, the second part is unlikely to get any marks. The answers to the second part are contingent on the first.

THE ORAL AND CLINICAL EXAMINATIONS

This is the crucial part of the examination and many candidates falter at this stage. Having reached this stage, your *PREPARATION* must be intensified. Know what is expected of a candidate in each part of the clinicals. The oral and clinical examinations are held on the same day and you will be examined by a different pair of examiners each time. As you have to 'sell' yourself in this part of the examination, do dress smartly and sensibly. Do not overdose with cologne or perfume but do not emanate other odours. Look professional at all times.

The oral examination

A pair of examiners will examine you for 20 minutes. Each examiner will question you for 10 minutes on at least three topics. Topics include management of common medical problems and emergencies, neonatology, current topics, basic applied physiology and basic statistics. It is useful to read through the leading articles in recent journals. You may be given a complex clinical problem and asked to outline a plan for investigations and management.

- Always think before you speak.
- Do not mention conditions that you know little about. Do not help the examiners in exposing your ignorance!
- Always try to mention common things first. You will not impress the examiners by mentioning small-print stuff first.
- If you are asked a topic which you know absolutely nothing about, admit it! The examiners can then go on with the next question.
- Do not argue with the examiners!
- Lastly, speak audibly and confidently, sit comfortably and try to keep your hands in check.

The clinical examination

The clinicals are divided into two parts, the long case and short cases. A different pair of examiners will examine you in each part.

Long case

The time allocated is 1 hour. It is difficult to anticipate the possible type of cases one will get. However, long cases are usually 'cold cases' which are brought in for the examination. Hence they are usually children with chronic or ongoing diseases. This examination is to test the candidate's ability to:

- Take a thorough history.
- Conduct a complete physical examination.
- Formulate a diagnosis or differential diagnosis.
- Plan relevant investigations.
- Formulate a plan of management.

Advice

- Always give yourself 10–15 minutes before the allocated time is up to consolidate your thoughts. Try to anticipate the examiners' questions and be prepared with the answers.
- In your case presentation, adopt a *'problem-orientated approach.'* Examiners now expect and prefer this approach.
- Most long cases are 'cold cases' — i.e. patients brought in specially for the exam. As you are likely to be told the diagnosis by the patient, examiners tend to be less interested in the diagnosis but more interested in your appreciation of the problems of the case. So be prepared.

- Do not present all the negative or irrelevant parts of the history and examination. Just mention that it is normal or nothing to note. However, *do* mention negative findings that are relevant to the case.
- Try not to read from your notes. You will appear more impressive this way. Look at the examiners when you are presenting your history and findings. Refer to your notes only to check certain points which you may be uncertain of or have forgotten.
- If you get a difficult case which you have no idea of the diagnosis, don't panic. Go back to basics. List down the positive findings and relevant part of the history. Draw up a list of differential diagnoses. Think of any further useful investigations. If you still have no idea of the likely diagnosis, it is possible that a diagnosis has not been made yet!
- Finally, practise, practise and practise! In particular, practise your presentation.

Short case

More candidates fail in the short cases than in any part of the clinical examination. In the allocated time of 30 minutes, the candidate will be shown, hopefully, several short cases. Each examiner takes you for 15 minutes on two or three systems. This examination is to test the candidate's ability to:

- Perform a competent examination of a system.
- Elicit the physical signs.
- Interpret the findings.
- Handle patients and parents competently.

The examiners will be watching the candidate closely for poor technique or for failure to pay due care to the patients or their parents.

Advice

- Practise how to examine each system correctly. This should include examination of joints, gait, developmental assessment, eyes, squint and the skin.
- Listen carefully to the examiners' instructions and questions. If you are asked to 'listen to the heart', it means you should auscultate. If you are asked 'what is the diagnosis?', give the answer and do not give all your findings. If you are uncertain of the examiners' instructions, ask.
- Do not spend *too* long on each patient. The more cases you see, the more marks you are likely to get.
- Do not repeat/check your findings when you are sure; e.g. do not keep eliciting the knee jerk when you have already demonstrated it on your first attempt.
- The examiners' main concern is to assess your ability to elicit the correct physical sign accurately. The diagnosis is *NOT* important. So do not worry about a child with an odd facies when you have no idea of the diagnosis. You may be asked to examine only the abdomen or eyes, hence just describe your findings.

CASE HISTORIES

The examination paper consists usually of five questions which are to be answered in 55 minutes, Of the five questions, at least one will be a short case history, the others being full-length case histories. In the *short-case histories*, medical emergencies (including poisonings) and their management are common topics. The aims of this paper are to test the candidate's:

* ability to deduce from the presented information what are the important and unimportant findings;
* ability to decide if further information or investigations are required before a diagnosis is possible;
* ability to give the probable diagnoses in a given clinical situation;
* ability to plan further relevant investigations;
* ability to plan a course of management.

How to answer the questions

This paper is commonly referred to as 'Grey cases' so do not expect a crystal-clear history with data pointing to a single diagnosis. There is usually *more* than one answer to each part of the question. The approach to each question should be as follows:

1. Read the question *carefully* and *note* down what you think is the important information.
2. On the basis of what is given, *list* down all the differential diagnosis that you can think of.
3. Then *compare* your diagnosis with the relevant data that is given in the question; the *best* answer is the one which can explain most of the history and findings.
4. If only one answer is required, give only *one!* There are no extra marks awarded for more than the number of answers required.
5. When investigations are asked for, again, firstly list down all the investigations that you can think of. Then pick those that will *clearly point* towards or *confirm* the diagnosis. Certain investigations, such as 'full blood count; urea and electrolytes; microscopy and culture of urine' are considered as single answers.
6. Avoid using abbreviations, they may mean something different to the examiner (e.g. FBC, SXR, CDH).

DATA INTERPRETATION

This paper consists of 10 *compulsory* questions to be answered within 45 minutes. The paper is designed to test the candidate's ability to assess a set of results of investigations in a clinical situation. A brief history or a stem sentence is usually given.

Topics covered are wide ranging. Besides conventional biochemical, haematological data and ECGs, other subjects covered include audiograms, genetic tree, chromosome karyotyping, growth charts, developmental data, respiratory function data, cerebral spinal fluid results and cardiac catheterization data.

Candidates are expected to know the normal values and ranges of common biochemical and haematological tests. The normal ranges of less common tests are usually provided. Results of laboratory investigations are given in SI units.

Approach to the paper

- As the marking is on a graded scale, the approach to each question should be as advised under the section on 'Case histories'.
- Always try to answer *all* the questions.
- NB. Questions with essentially *normal* results can be expected.

PROJECTED MATERIAL

This part of the examination consists of 20 *compulsory* questions. Each question consists of a brief stem of one or two sentences and is based on a slide or pair of slides. The total time allocated is 40 minutes, i.e. 2 minutes per slide. Half a minute before each slide change, a visible (light) and audible (buzzer) warning will be given. There is *No* RE-RUN of the slides!

This paper is designed to test the candidate's ability:

- to identify (in a short time) a clinical condition, i.e. to give a diagnosis;
- to identify abnormalities;
- to suggest the appropriate investigation(s) and treatment.

Almost anything can come up in this paper. They include pictures of patients, blood films, CAT scans of brain, cranial ultrasound scans, pathological materials (CSF, biopsy materials). Pictures of *skin* and *eyes* are popular.

How to approach this paper

- See as many slides of as many different conditions as you can. A projected image of a condition can look quite different because of the magnification.
- If you don't have anyone to show you slides, the next best thing to do is to go through the photographs in as many major paediatric textbooks or atlases as you can find in your local medical library.
- *Read* the stem sentence(s) and the question carefully before answering. Many candidates only look at the slide and then answer without due attention to the question. The question may ask for the abnormality rather than the diagnosis.
- Be specific — if a lesion is on the left, state so. Otherwise you are likely to be marked down.

DIPLOMA IN CHILD HEALTH EXAMINATION (LONDON)

Each of the London, Glasgow and Dublin Colleges hold their own DCH examination and candidates are advised to seek details from the appropriate college.

THE WRITTEN SECTION

This section consists of two papers.

Written Paper I (3 hours)

This paper consists of (a) 20 short note questions, and (b) two case histories.

(a) Short note questions
These consist of 50% of the total marks. Any subject matter may be asked. With the current emphasis on community and social paediatrics, candidates are well advised to read up on these topics. All the questions require precise and concise answers.

- Write in short sentences.
- Space out and use *headings*. This helps the examiner in the marking and you are likely to score more marks.
- Write legibly. Remember that the examiner has a pile of question papers to mark.

(b) Case histories
There are two case histories, each of which carry 25% of the marks. The case histories are in a similar vein as those in the MRCP examination but perhaps slightly less 'grey'. The histories are orientated towards cases presented to a GP surgery. There are usually fewer laboratory investigations to interpret.

- Read the history carefully (see section under case histories).
- Answer the question concisely. Some questions may require a few *short* sentences.

Written Paper 2 (2 hours)

This paper consists of 60 multiple choice questions with five parts to each. Remember the importance of this paper — you can proceed to the clinical examinations only if you achieved a pass in this paper. See the section under Multiple Choice Questions.

THE CLINICAL EXAMINATION

There have been significant recent changes to the format and composition of the clinical examination. It is advisable to obtain the

most recent information regarding the regulations and syllabus
from the London Royal College.

There are three pairs of examiners in the clinical section. One
pair will have marked your Written Paper 1, another pair will take
you on the long case, and the last pair will examine you on the
short cases. It is a fair examination!

Long case

You are assigned a patient for 40 minutes during which you have to
take a history, examine the patient, and you will be expected to be
able to define any clinical and social problems, and be able to make
a diagnosis and plan the management. Patients without clinical
signs will have a good history. You then spend 20 minutes with the
examiners. Read the guidelines under the MRCP section.

Short cases

The total time allocated is 25 minutes of which 10 minutes will be
devoted to developmental assessment, including the testing of
vision, for squint (cover test) and hearing. It is particularly
important that candidates are familiar and competent with the
developmental assessment of young children.

The short cases are designed to test the candidates' ability to:

- examine children competently;
- examine each system and elicit physical signs;
- assess the clinical significance of their findings;
- plan a course of investigations and management;
- the diagnosis is less important than your ability to elicit physical
  signs accurately.

Candidates should remember that minor surgical and orthopaedic
cases may also be presented in this examination.

MARKING SYSTEM

Each pair of examiners will award a mark ranging from 0–10 for
each part of the examination, i.e. Paper 1, Long case and Short
case. An aggregate mark of 15 is required to pass. However, in
order to pass, a candidate must achieve at least a 5 in each of the
Long and Short cases.

MULTIPLE CHOICE EXAMINATION

This examination is designed to test the breadth of the candidate's
knowledge of general paediatrics. The questions are designed to
contain no ambiguities and no hidden traps! In the DCH
examination, the MCQ examination serves as a screening test. Only
candidates who have achieved a certain pass mark will be invited
to attend the clinicals. The pass mark is not known but as the

number of centres which will be holding the clinicals are predetermined, it is unlikely that the number of candidates for the clinicals will exceed that which can be accommodated by the clinical centres. The mark obtained in the MCQ examination *will not* be carried forward to the clinical examination.

How to prepare and approach the paper

- Read as extensively as you can. While doing so, try to think how the facts can be asked in a MCQ.
- Practise doing MCQ as often as you can. Try to identify your weak subjects and then read up on them.

In the examination:

- Read the instructions and questions carefully. Make sure you know how to mark your answers on the answer sheet.
- Answer first those questions that you know well.
- Do not guess if you have absolutely no knowledge of any question.
- Make an informed deduction on those questions which you have some knowledge. Work from first principles if necessary.
- If you finish ahead of time, do not spend too much time going over your answers. You may become confused.
- Although it is not advisable to count the number of questions you have answered and the score you may get, it is true to say that you are unlikely to pass if you have left too many questions unanswered.

Reference

Anderson J. How to tackle multiple choice questions papers. Hospital Update 1982; 8: 593–596

II Case histories

A 10-year-old Rastafarian girl was admitted to hospital because of increasing abdominal discomfort and pain. She was one of 4 siblings and the family lived closely among other Rastafarians. The girl had been listless and anorexic for the past few weeks. She had no bowel symptoms.

Examination revealed a pleasant girl. Her height and weight were on the 50th centile. She had a low-grade fever, 37.9°C. Other than mild pharyngitis, the examination of the respiratory system was normal. Her abdomen was distended with a discernible fluid thrill. Liver and spleen were not palpable. The rest of the physical examination was normal. Urinalysis showed a trace of protein but no glucose or blood. Microscopy was normal.

Investigations

Haemoglobin 10 g/dl
WBC 12.5 × 10⁹/l
ESR 86 mm/1st hour
Serum urea 4.4 mmol/l
Serum creatinine 48 μmol/l
Total serum protein 59 g/l
Serum albumin 26 g/l
Serum Aspartate transaminase 37 iu/l
Serum total bilirubin 15 μmol/l
Chest X-ray normal
Electrocardiogram normal

A What is the most likely diagnosis?
B What two investigations would be most helpful in this case?

Answer to question 1

A +4   Abdominal tuberculosis.
   +3   Malignant disease.
   +1   Chronic liver disease with ascites.
   +1   Nephrotic syndrome.
   +1   Budd–Chiari syndrome.
   0   Constructive pericarditis.
   0   Heart failure.

B +3   Mantoux test 1:10 000 followed by 1:1000.
   +3   Diagnostic paracentesis — stain fluid for acid and alcohol fast bacilli and culture (AAFB).
   +3   Three early gastric washings — stain for AAFB and culture.
   +1   Measure protein content of ascitic fluid.
   +1   Cell cytology of ascitic fluid.
   0   Abdominal X-ray.
   0   Abdominal ultrasound.

Maximum marks +10

The 4-week history of listlessness and anorexia, Rastafarian background, high ESR and absence of any clear evidence of hepatic, renal and cardiac data, make abdominal tuberculosis the best possible answer. Malignancy obviously cannot be excluded. Nephrotic syndrome is only vaguely suggested on the basis of a low serum albumin and the urine contained only a trace of protein which would be unusual. Chronic liver disease is a possibility. Such a patient would have low serum albumin, but the serum aspartate transaminase is normal and is not a good marker of chronic liver disease. The prothrombin test is better. Budd–Chiari syndrome is produced by obstruction to the hepatic vein. The obstruction is due to a variety of causes. It may present with abdominal pain and vomiting, marked and tender hepatomegaly, ascites (usually blood-stained) and mild jaundice.

Question 2

A 10-year-old schoolboy was referred to hospital. He was an active boy and played football and rugby for his school. Four months ago he complained of a sore neck, shoulders and knees. He thought that his symptoms might be related to his sporting activities. However, 2 weeks ago he had a sore throat and fever, and again complained of a sore neck and pains in his knees and right elbow. He was seen by his family doctor who diagnosed tonsillitis and prescribed a course of oral ampicillin and paracetamol. His fever and sore throat resolved after 2 days but he continued to complain of pain in his knees.

He had a younger sister aged 8. She was well. However, his father suffered from psoriasis. The birth history was normal.

On examination he was found to be a quiet boy. His temperature was 37°C. There was no skin rash. His tonsils were not inflamed. However, a few cervical nodes were palpable. His heart rate was 86/minute and his blood pressure was 98/60. There was a soft short systolic murmur best heard in the lower left sternal edge. The second heart sound was normal. Both knees were slightly swollen and there was an effusion in the left knee. Movements were restricted. The rest of the examination was normal. Urine analysis showed no protein, blood or cells.

Investigations

Haemoglobin 10.9 g/dl
WBC 8.2 × 10⁹/l

A What is the most likely diagnosis?
B What is the significance of the heart murmur?
C Give three further investigations that would help most in the diagnosis.

Answer to question 2

A +3 Juvenile chronic arthritis or juvenile rheumatoid arthritis.
    +3 Still's disease.
    +3 Pauci-articular juvenile chronic arthritis.
    +1 Glandular fever.
    +1 Psoriatic juvenile chronic arthritis.
    0 Rheumatic fever.
    0 Subacute bacterial endocarditis.
    0 Trauma.

B +2 Innocent or benign murmur.
    +1 Small ventricular septal defect.
    0 Mitral valve prolapse.
    0 Subacute bacterial endocarditis.

C +2 X-rays of knees, elbows, shoulders and neck.
    +2 Rheumatoid factor.
    +2 Antinuclear factor.
    +2 ESR.
    +2 C-reactive protein.
    +2 Slit-lamp examination of uveitis.
    +2 Monospot/Paul–Bunnell.

Maximum marks +11

The relevant information is the chronicity and the recurring history of joint pains and fever. Together with the findings of minimal lymphadenopathy and swollen joints, the best answer is juvenile chronic arthritis. Glandular fever is a possibility but the course of ampicillin treatment might have precipitated the typical rash. There are no diagnostic tests to confirm juvenile chronic arthritis.

Question 3

A 6-year-old boy was admitted to hospital following a generalised convulsion. He had been unwell for 2 days with headaches, vomiting and some visual disturbances. He also suffers from primary nocturnal enuresis. However, because he drinks a lot of fluid and hence passes much urine, his mother had restricted his fluid intake in the previous few days. He was an only child and the birth history was unremarkable.

On examination he was semicomatose, responsive only to painful stimuli. His temperature was 37°C. Fundoscopy showed no papilloedema although there was a small retinal haemorrhage in the right eye. The apex beat was forceful but not displaced. There were no murmurs. His blood pressure was 170/110. There was no meningism or any focal neurological signs. Urine analysis showed pH 7, protein +++, trace glucose. Shortly after admission, he had a further convulsion.

A   What is the most likely diagnosis?
B   What important therapeutic step would you take (besides stopping the convulsion)?
C   Give two investigations that are most helpful in the further management?

Answer to question 3

A +4 Acute hypertensive encephalopathy secondary to underlying renal disease.
     +2 Hypertension.
     +2 Chronic renal failure.
     +2 Cerebrovascular accident.
     0   Afebrile convulsion.
     0   Intracerebral tumours.
     0   Meningitis.

B +2 Antihypertensive therapy.
     +2 Intravenous hydralazine, diazoxide or labetalol.
     0   Intravenous fluid or IV drip.

C +2 Serum creatinine.
     +2 Assess glomerular filtration rate.
     +2 Renal ultrasound.
     +2 Renal biopsy.
     +1 Urea and electrolytes.

Maximum marks +10

The child has suffered a convulsion due to acute hypertensive encephalopathy. The history of polyuria and polydipsia and raised blood pressure with proteinuria are strongly suggestive of a chronic renal problem. Other answers are not precise enough.

In the management it is important to control the blood pressure and it should be lowered slowly to around 90 mm diastolic. Further investigations should include tests that would confirm a chronic renal problem and clarify the pathology.

Question 4

A 2-month-old female infant referred to hospital because of pallor. She was well till 3 weeks ago when she developed an episode of vomiting and diarrhoea. She was visited by her family doctor who prescribed Dioralyte (dextrose-electrolyte solution). Her diarrhoea stopped after 48 hours and she was better by the fourth day. However, her feeding remained somewhat poorly and she saw her family doctor again. She was noticed to be pale but the mother said her baby has always looked like that. She is the second child of unrelated, healthy Caucasian parents. She was born at term by normal delivery. She had mild jaundice but did not require phototherapy. She was breast fed for the first 4 weeks and then onto bottle feeding.

On examination she was found to be a well-nourished infant. Her temperature was 37°C. Her weight, length and head circumference were all around the 50th percentile. She looked pale. There was no petechia or bruises. The liver edge was palpable 2 cm below the right costal margin. The spleen was just tipped. The examination of the cardiovascular, respiratory and central nervous system was normal. Urine analysis showed no bile, urobilinogen, protein or glucose.

The following investigations were done after admission:

Haemoglobin 6.5 g/dl
WBC 10.2 × 10^9/l
Platelets 200 × 10^9/dl
MCV 95 fl
Reticulocyte count 0.5%
Coombs' test negative
Serum iron 17 μmol/l
Serum iron binding capacity 65 μmol/l
Serum B$_{12}$ and folate normal
Bone marrow smear showed normal cellularity, myeloid and megakaryocyte series. Reduced normoblasts

What is the most likely diagnosis?

Answer to question 4

+5   Congenital hypoplastic anaemia or pure red cell aplasia or
     Diamond–Blackfan syndrome.
+4   Aplastic crisis resolving.
+2   Fanconi's anaemia.
+2   Late anaemia of haemolytic disease of the newborn.
0   Haemolytic anaemia.
0   Congenital spherocytosis.

Total marks +5

The key to the diagnosis is the bone marrow smear which showed
mainly diminished red blood cell precursors. Although this may
also occur in a resolving episode of aplastic crisis, but taking into
account the long history of pallor, the diagnosis of congenital pure
red cell aplasia is most likely. In Fanconi's anaemia, the white cell
and platelet counts are also depressed although pancytopenia is
not usually present at birth or during early infancy. Furthermore,
some two-thirds of affected children have other associated
congenital anomalies.

The late anaemia of haemolytic disease of the newborn is a
possible diagnosis. However, in such a case one would have a clear
neonatal history and the Rhesus status of mother and infant would
have been known.

A diagnosis of haemolytic anaemia (or other conditions causing
it) is not acceptable as it is too vague. Furthermore, the reticulocyte count, urine analysis and bone marrow results do not
support the diagnosis in any way.

Question 5

A boy was born by forceps delivery at term to a 28-year-old primigravida. The labour was essentially uneventful except for two brief episodes of Type II dips about 1 hour prior to delivery. At birth he was noted to be cyanosed and had poor tone. He gasped twice. The attending midwife then applied face-mask ventilation while the paediatrician was called. On the paediatrician's arrival, he found a well-grown term infant who looked slightly pale with central cyanosis. His respiration was irregular and the chest was overinflated. The heart rate was 110/min. The heart sounds on the left were present but soft. Air entry was better heard on the right side. The liver and spleen were not palpable.

A What is the most likely diagnosis?
B Give three other immediate procedures that you would perform.

Answer to question 5

A +4 Congenital diaphragmatic hernia or left diaphragmatic hernia (with birth asphyxia).
+4 Birth asphyxia.
+1 Left pneumothorax.
+1 Cyanotic heart disease.
0   Inadequate resuscitation.
0   Meconium aspiration.

B +2 Intubate and apply intermittent positive ventilation.
+2 Pass a thick-bore nasogastric tube.
+2 Correct acidosis (± hypoglycaemia).
+2 Check acid−base status.
+1 Chest X-ray.
+1 Electrocardiogram.
+1 Echocardiogram.

Total marks +10

This question is designed to test the candidate's ability to deal with a neonatal emergency. The initial history is suggestive of an intrapartum hypoxic event and a 'shocked' floppy baby is suggestive of birth asphyxia. However, the persistent cyanosis, overinflated chest, diminished air entry and 'soft' heart sounds on the left should make one think of a diaphragmatic hernia. Auscultation of heart sounds on the right would be essential.

Left pneumothorax is not a good answer as it has ignored the other features mentioned. Cyanotic heart disease rarely presents at birth.

The immediate procedures should be directed at resuscitating the infant and correcting hypoxia and metabolic disturbance. When these are done, diagnostic procedures can follow.

Question 6

A 3-month-old male Caucasian infant was admitted as an emergency with a history of persistent, bile-stained vomiting. He was found to have a strangulated inguinal hernia on laparotomy and 5 cm (2″) of the small bowel had to be resected. Postoperatively, he developed severe salmonella gastroenteritis and had torrential diarrhoea. He was transferred to the Regional Gastroenteritis Unit for continuing care and total parenteral nutrition (TPN).

On examination his temperature was 37.2°C and mildly dehydrated. Heart sounds were normal. Liver was palpable 2 cm below the right costal margin.

A Silastic catheter was inserted via a peripheral vein into the superior vena cava and he was started on parenteral feeding (TPN) using Vamin/dextrose and Intralipid 10% solutions.

On the tenth day following TPN, he developed a temperature of 38°C. Culture of blood and catheter site showed a growth of Candida albicans. Anti-fungal treatment was given intravenously for a total of 10 days. Two days after starting treatment, the temperature settled and he was clinically better.

On day 17, a grade 2/6 systolic murmur was noted over the pulmonary area. On the 25th day, he was noted to be unwell and jaundiced; the spleen was palpable 2 cm and the liver was 4 cm below the costal margins.

Investigations at this point showed:

Haemoglobin 10.5 g/dl
WBC 18 × 10⁹/1
Platelets 94 × 10⁹/1
SGOT 158 iu/l
SGPT 140 iu/l
Total bilirubin 148 μmol/l
Direct bilirubin 110 μmol/l

Urinalysis showed a trace of protein, blood, urobilinogen but no glucose. Microscopy revealed no cells or organisms.

A What is the most likely cause for the infant's deterioration?
B Give two investigations that would be most useful in this case.

Answer to question 6

A +4 *Candida albicans* endocarditis.
   +4 Fungal endocarditis.
   +4 Subacute endocarditis.
   +1 Septicaemia.
   +1 Haemolysis.
   +1 Disseminated intravascular coagulation.
   0   Hepatitis.

B +3 Series of blood cultures.
   +3 Echocardiography.
   +1 Blood culture.
   +1 Clotting studies.

Total marks +10

The emergence of a murmur, the presence of haemolysis, haematuria, splenomegaly and the history of a candida fungaemia in an unwell child are suggestive of candida endocarditis. A diagnosis of hepatitis is too vague. Furthermore, the liver transaminases were not grossly elevated. In suspected subacute bacterial endocarditis, a series rather than single blood culture should be done.

Question 7

A 2-year-old girl was brought by her mother to the Casualty Department during the early hours of the morning because she had a convulsion.

Examination showed a thin child who was irritable when roused. The temperature was 37.3°C. There were some bruises on her legs and shoulders. Fundoscopy showed some retinal haemorrhages in the right eye. The mother said the bruises were sustained a week ago when the child fell down the stairs.

X-ray of the skull and long bones were normal. One hour after admission to hospital, she had another convulsion which was rapidly controlled with intravenous diazepam.

A   What is the most likely diagnosis?
B   What immediate test would you do next to confirm your diagnosis?

Answer to question 7

A +4 Subdural haematoma secondary to excessive shaking.
+4 Intracranial haemorrhage due to non-accidental injury.
+3 Intracranial bleeding.
+3 Non-accidental injury.
0   Idiopathic thrombocytopenic purpura.

B +3 CAT scan of brain.
+1 Clotting studies.
+1 Skeletal survey.
0   Photographs.
0   Full blood count.

Total marks +7

The presence of bruises and retinal haemorrhages should point towards non-accidental injury. As no blood result was given, a diagnosis of idiopathic thrombocytopenic purpura cannot be accepted.

An intracranial bleeding should be confirmed by a CAT scan of the brain. Other tests to support the diagnosis of non-accidental injury are done subsequently.

Question 8

A 28-year-old primigravida gave birth to a female infant at 38 weeks gestation. The mother had polyhydramnios and mild pre-eclampsia during pregnancy. The infant was born by normal vaginal delivery and weighed 2.8 kg. At birth, the infant failed to establish spontaneous respiration and required intubation and subsequently ventilation. There was no monitoring during labour but the fetal heart rate some 30 minutes before birth was recorded as normal.

Examination revealed a floppy and oedematous infant. She had bilateral club feet. There were very little facial movements. Knee jerks were elicited. The examination of the cardiovascular, respiratory and gastrointestinal system was normal. The infant required assisted ventilation for about 21 days. She was tube fed for about 2 months.

Results of investigations were:

Haemoglobin 15 g/dl
Serum urea and electrolytes normal
Blood sugar normal
Urine and plasma amino-acid profile normal
Cranial ultrasound normal
Electroencephalogram normal
CAT scan of brain normal
Chromosomal karyotype 46XX

A   What is the most likely diagnosis?
B   What two tests would you do that would give you the most information?

Answer to question 8

A   +5   Neonatal myotonic dystrophica.
+4   Wernig–Hoffman disease (infantile spinal muscular atrophy).
+4   Congenital muscular dystrophy.
+3   Neonatal (transient) myasthenia gravis.
+1   Spinal cord trauma.
+1   Myotonia congenita.
0   Duchenne's muscular dystrophy.

B   +2   Examine the mother for facial weakness, myotonic grip. Percussion of thenar eminence. Demonstrate the inability to bury the lower eyelashes when closing her eyes.
+2   Electromyography in mother.
+2   Muscle biopsy.
+2   Tensilon (edrophonium chloride) test.
+1   Nerve conduction studies.
+1   Creatine kinase.

Total marks +9

This case consists of information that is characteristic of neonatal myotonic dystrophica which is an autosomal dominant condition. The important features were extreme hypotonia, oedema, history of polyhydramnios, little respiratory effort at birth, joint deformities and facial diplegia in neonatal form. The mother is always affected. In Wernig–Hoffman disease, fibrillations in the tongue may be present. Tendon reflexes are usually absent. Muscle biopsy shows atrophic changes. Congenital muscular dystrophy is an autosomal recessive condition. It is difficult to differentiate from Wernig–Hoffman disease. Fibrillations are absent and tendon jerks are present but depressed. Muscle enzymes are normal but biopsy shows dystrophic changes. In neonatal myasthenia gravis (transient), there is usually a positive maternal history. The tensilon test is diagnostic.

Tests like nerve conduction studies and creatine kinase are generally less helpful and are usually normal in the above conditions.

Question 9

A 3-week-old neonate was referred to the hospital because of poor feeding and rapid breathing. She had been feeding well till that day. She was born at term by normal delivery, weighing 3.2 kg.

On examination, she was a well-grown, restless and pale baby. Her temperature was 37.4°C. She had a clear nasal discharge. Both tympanic membranes and the throat were slightly pink. The anterior fontanelle was soft. The respiratory rate was 45/minute with minimal costal recession. The heart rate was more than 200/minute. The liver was 2 cm below the right costal margin. The rest of the examination was normal.

An ECG showed a supraventricular tachycardia with a rate of 280/min.

A   What immediate therapeutic step would you take?
B   Suggest two other therapeutic measures you would take if the initial one failed.

Answer to question 9

A +2 Carotid sinus massage (one side at a time).
    +2 Ice-pack to face.
    +2 Eyeball pressure.

B +2 Intravenous verapamil.
    +2 Digoxin.
    +2 Cardioversion.

Maximum marks +6

This question tests the candidate's ability to deal with a cardiac emergency.

Supraventricular tachycardia is of abrupt onset and is often precipitated by an acute infection. The attack may stop abruptly without treatment. Prolonged attacks should be stopped because they lead to cardiac discomfort and congestive heart failure.

Vagal stimulation like unilateral carotid sinus massage may abort the attack. Eyeball pressure should be done cautiously because of potential eye injury. The diving reflex can be elicited by applying cold ice packs or a flannel to the face. Older children could be taught various vago-tonic manoeuvres.

If cardiac failure is present then cardioversion is recommended. Drug treatment with intravenous verapamil, digoxin and propranol are also effective.

Question 10

A 2-year-old child was brought up to the Accident and Emergency Department after having been found semi-comatose. There were some tablets found near him and the tablets were prescribed for his father who has some diarrhoea.

On examination he was semi-comatose responding to painful stimuli. He looked flushed, temperature 38.5°C, and had a dry mouth. Both pupils were constricted. Muscle tone was diminished with sluggish tendon reflexes. Respiration rate was 60/min, heart rate 148/min.

A   What is the most likely diagnosis?
B   Give two therapeutic measures which may be useful to alleviate some of the symptoms.

Answer to question 10

A +4 Lomotil poisoning — it contains diphenoxylate
hydrochloride (an opiate) and atropine sulphate.

B +2 Intravenous naloxone — to reverse opiate effects.
+2 Pilocarpine — for peripheral effects of atropine.
+2 Airway — ventilation.

Maximum marks +8

Lomotil is commonly prescribed for the treatment of diarrhoea in
adults. The clinical features are typical of Lomotil poisoning.

The small pupils and central depression are due to the opiate
effects of diphenoxylate hydrochloride. This could be reversed
by administering naloxone intravenously.

The fever, flushed cheeks, dry mouth and often urine retention
are due to the atropine effects. Giving pilocarpine may reverse only
the peripheral effects. If the child remains centrally depressed and
if respiration is compromised, then assisted ventilation may be
required.

Question 11

A 10-year-old boy was referred to hospital with a 2-month history of central abdominal pain which was associated with three episodes of vomiting small amounts of blood. He has been generally unwell with poor appetite and weight loss for several months. A few weeks prior to admission, he developed some pruritus. He is the eldest of three siblings and parents are healthy and there is no consanguinity. The birth history was normal and so was his development. He had been treated for iron deficiency anaemia 3 years ago. It was also noted in school that his work has fallen off over the past few terms.

Examination revealed a thin, unwell, pale and icteric boy. Temperature was 37°C. Blood pressure was 105/70. The liver was 4 cm below the right costal margin and the spleen was not palpable. Fundal examination showed normal optic discs. Other than some weakness of his limbs and ankle oedema, the rest of the examination was normal. Urine analysis showed protein +, blood + and glucose +.

Results of investigations were:

Haemoglobin 7.6 g/dl
WBC 11.6 × 10⁹/l
Platelets 200 × 10⁹/l
Blood film — occasional target cells
Coombs' test negative
Serum bilirubin 58 μmol/l
SGOT 120 iu/l
Alkaline phosphatase 571 iu/l
Albumin 20 g/l
Serum creatinine 55 μmol/l
Prothrombin time 37 s/control 13 s
HBsAg and hepatitis A serology negative
Serum hepatoglobins not detectable

A What is the most likely diagnosis?
B What two investigations would be most useful to confirm your diagnosis?

Answer to question 11

A +4 Wilson's disease (hepatolenticular degeneration).
   +2 Chronic liver disease.
   0   Hepatitis.

B +2 Slit-lamp examination of eyes for Kayser–Fleischer rings.
   +2 Serum caeruloplasmin.
   +2 24 hour urine collection for copper concentration.
   +2 Liver biopsy to assay copper content.
   +1 Serum copper level.
   +1 Liver biopsy.

Total marks +10

The presence of acute haemolysis, hepatic disorder, intellectual impairment and renal tubular damage are highly suggestive of Wilson's disease. The diagnosis of chronic liver disease is less specific and hence will get less marks.

Of the tests listed, checking serum copper level is usually unhelpful. It can be low, normal or high. When liver biopsy is listed as an investigation, it is desirable to be more specific.

Question 12

A 5-year-old boy was referred to the outpatient clinic. About 8 weeks ago he was seen in the Accident and Emergency Unit following a fall in school on a snowy day. He sustained a small haematoma on his head and some abrasions on his arms and legs. There were no fractures. However, since then he has been noted to be slightly unsteady when he walks. His parents had noted this prior to the accident but did not think it was as bad. His school teacher had also remarked that he was not good at gym and cannot run.

He is the youngest of three children, his two sisters are aged 9 and 11 years and both are well. Both parents are healthy. He was born at term by normal delivery. He was in the Special Care Baby Unit because of jaundice which required 3 days phototherapy. He sat up unaided at 7 months and walked at 14 months. He spoke a few words by 1 year and sentences by 2 years.

Examination revealed a quiet boy. He was well built and both height and weight were just below the 50th percentile. The temperature was 37°C. His heart rate was 100/min and blood pressure 80/54. There were no audible murmurs. The examination of the gastrointestinal and respiratory system was normal. The cranial nerves examination was normal. Muscle tone in all limbs were normal but the power was diminished. Knee tendon reflexes were absent and the plantar reflexes were flexor. He walked on tiptoes. He had a lumbar lordosis. Both tendon Achilles were tight and there was bilateral pes cavus. Sensory testing was normal.

A What is the most likely diagnosis?
B Give two investigations that would be most helpful in confirming the diagnosis.

Answer to question 12

A +4 Duchenne muscular dystrophy.
   +2 Muscular dystrophy (or scapuloperoneal, limb girdle, Becker).
   +1 Friedreich's ataxia.
   0   Trauma.
   0   Perthes' disease.
   0   Cerebral palsy.

B +2 Serum creatine phosphokinase.
   +2 Muscle biopsy.
   +2 Electromyography.
   0   Nerve conduction study.

Maximum marks +10

Important features to be noted in the history are: the abnormality in walking at home and in school, unable to run, marginally slow in walking, well-built boy, somewhat fast heart rate, diminished power, walking on tip-toes, lordosis, bilateral pes cavus and absent knee jerks. All these point towards Duchenne muscular dystrophy. Some of the other forms of muscular dystrophy share some similarities. In Friedreich's ataxia, there are more pyramidal signs with loss of joint position and vibration sense. There is also often ataxia of upper limbs with intention tremor. Speech is also affected.

Investigations to confirm the diagnosis must include the three listed above. The serum creatine phosphokinase level is grossly elevated. The electromyogram shows myopathic changes. Muscle biopsy shows typical rounded opaque muscle fibres scattered throughout. Ultrasound examination of muscle group is used only in a few very specialized centres. Nerve conduction study is unhelpful.

Question 13

A 1-year-old infant was brought to the Accident and Emergency Unit one afternoon because he had suddenly become very 'blue'. He had been followed up by another hospital because of a heart defect. The mother said the child was usually pink but did become dusky at times, especially when he cried. He has had two previous brief episodes. No previous operations have been done. There was no history of choking or inhalation of foreign body.

Examination revealed a semi-comatose and deeply cyanosed infant. Respirations were rapid and shallow.

A What three immediate therapeutic measures would you take in this case?

B What is the diagnosis?

Answer to question 13

A +2 Oxygen by face-mask.
+2 Place child in chest-knee position.
+2 Intravenous morphine or propranolol.
+2 Correct metabolic acidosis.

B +4 Acute cyanotic attack — Fallot's tetralogy.

Maximum marks +10

Paroxysmal cyanotic attacks are well-recognized problems in children with Fallot's tetralogy. They are common in the first couple of years of life. The attack occurs frequently in the morning and can last from a few minutes to a few hours. Occasionally it may be fatal.

The attacks are due to a reduction of pulmonary blood flow which leads to hypoxia and metabolic acidosis. This decrease in pulmonary blood flow will also lead to an increase in the right to left shunting. Resuscitative measures should be directed at decreasing systemic venous return, preventing hypoxia, correcting metabolic acidosis and drugs to reverse the infundibular spasm.

Question 14

A male infant, the first child of unrelated parents, was born at full term by normal delivery. The birth weight was 3.4 kg, and Apgar score at 1 minute was 8. On the second day he was noted to be slightly icteric but he was feeding well. At the age of 56 hours, he was noted to be cold and had peripheral cyanosis.

On examination, he was floppy and centrally cyanosed. Temperature was 35.9°C. The fontanelle was soft. Respiratory rate was 68/min and breath sounds were vesicular with equal air entry on both sides. Peripheral pulses were thready and difficult to feel. There was no heart murmur. The liver was 4 cm below the right costal margin. The spleen was not palpable.

Investigations

Haemoglobin 18 g/dl
WBC $13.0 \times 10^9/l$
Platelets $350 \times 10^9/l$
Sodium 135 mmol/l
Potassium 4.0 mmol/l
Urea 4 mmol/l
Blood sugar 0.5 mmol/l
Arterial blood gases: pH 6.98, P_{O_2}, 6.5 kPa, P_{CO_2}, 5.1 kPa, BE-20 in 90% oxygen

A   What is the most likely diagnosis?
B   Give three further investigations that would be most helpful in this case.

Answer to question 14

A +4 Hypoplastic left heart syndrome.
   +4 Septicaemia.
   +1 Transposition of the great vessels.
   0 Congenital heart disease.
   0 Hypoglycaemia.

B +2 Blood culture.
   +2 Lumbar puncture.
   +2 Echocardiography.
   +2 Cardiac catheterization.
   +2 Chest X-ray.

Maximum marks +10

The history strongly implies that the infant is very ill. The clinical signs suggest either sepsis or a congenital heart lesion like hypoplastic left heart syndrome. In this condition, heart failure is the early presentation. The infant is dyspnoeic, liver is enlarged and peripheral pulses are weak or absent. The heart is enlarged. The infant often has a greyish blue colour. Echocardiogram is diagnostic and it shows gross abnormalities of the left heart structures. Cardiac catheterization is useful but is being superceded by echocardiography.

Transposition of the great vessel usually present with cyanosis shortly after birth. Only if early signs are ignored would the infant then give the picture as described above.

Hypoglycaemia is a common finding in a sick neonate. It is not a diagnosis and the cause of the hypoglycaemia should be ascertained.

Blood culture and lumbar puncture are required to look for the source of sepsis. A chest X-ray would also demonstrate cardiomegaly and any lung pathology.

Question 15

A 12-year-old Indian boy was referred to hospital with a history of difficulty in walking. He was the youngest of five siblings who were all well. He had arrived in England only 4 days previously. He had been well till about 4 weeks previously when he developed a fever, sore throat, headache and some vomiting. He was seen by a local doctor and was given an injection. He felt better 2 days later and was able to attend school. Because of his imminent trip to England, he and his parents had been travelling a lot to see and visit their relatives. He said that he had felt unduly tired with all these activities. On a few occasions he had 'collapsed' and 'his legs felt weak suddenly'. Soon after he arrived in England, he had not been well and complained of shortness of breath.

He was born at term at home. There were no neonatal problems. He had had no immunizations. Examination revealed a thin boy. He looked clinically anaemic. His temperature was 37.2°C. The heart rate was 90/min and blood pressure was 100/70. His chest expansion was equal and air entry was good. His respiratory rate was 24/min. Fundoscopy showed normal optic discs. The muscle tone and power in the lower limbs were decreased. There was some wasting of calf and quadricep muscles in both legs. The knee and ankle jerks were absent. Touch and pain sensations were intact. Both plantars were flexor. Urine analysis showed no protein, blood or glucose.

A   What is the most likely diagnosis?
B   Give two investigations that are most likely to provide diagnostic information.

Answer to question 15

A +4 Poliomyelitis.
   +4 Guillain-Barré syndrome (acute infective polyneuritis).
   +1 Acute porphyria.
   0   Muscular dystrophy of any type.

B +3 Isolation of poliovirus from stools or throat.
   +3 Lumbar puncture to determine cell count and protein
        content.
   +3 Peripheral nerve conduction study.
   +3 Paired viral titres.
   +2 Isolation of poliovirus from CSF.
   0   Blood cultures.

Maximum marks +10

The history of a febrile illness followed by weakness in the legs,
difficulty with walking and shortness of breath should point
towards an infective/neurological problem. Furthermore, the lack
of previous immunizations and the clinical findings of a lower
motor neuron lesion should make poliomyelitis or acute infective
polyneuritis the two best possible diagnoses. Poliomyelitis is rare
in the UK with a routine immunization programme. In both
conditions, a preceding history of a febrile illness is common. The
outcome in poliomyelitis is variable and different systems may be
affected. In acute infective polyneuritis the onset of weakness may
be sudden. The weakness is symmetrical and the lower limbs and
distal muscles are most severely affected.
   In both conditions there is hypotonia and hyporeflexia. Sensory
involvement is usually minimal or absent. Respiration can be
affected in either condition. In poliomyelitis, the virus can be
isolated from the throat during the early stages of the illness. It can
be found in the stools for many weeks after onset. The virus is not
often isolated from the CSF. The CSF will show a mild pleocytosis
with slight to moderate rise in protein content. However, in acute
infective polyneuritis the cell count is normal but the protein is
markedly raised. Nerve conduction study shows a decrease in
conduction velocity.

Question 16

A girl weighing 3.8 kg was born at 40 weeks to a 28-year-old mother following a difficult vaginal delivery because of shoulder dystocia. The Apgars were 4 at 1 min, 8 at 10 minutes and the infant required some oxygen given by face-mask for about 3 minutes. The membranes had been ruptured 18 hours previously and mother had a temperature of 38°C during the later part of her labour. At birth the infant was noted to have little movement of the right arm except the fingers. At 1 hour old the infant was noted to have a respiratory rate of 80/min recession. There were no other abnormal signs. Results of initial investigations were:

Haemoglobin 15.8 g/dl
Corrected white cell count 12 × 10⁹/l
Arterial blood gases in 28% O_2 pH 7.25
P_{CO_2} 5.8 kPa
P_{O_2} 7.2 kPa
BM test (for glucose) 2.2 mmol/l

A What is the most likely cause of the tachypnoea?
B Give two investigations which will be most helpful in this case.

Answer to question 16

A +4 Congenital pneumonia.
   +4 Sepsis (e.g. Group B streptococcal infection).
   +4 Spontaneous pneumothorax.
   +4 Phrenic nerve palsy.
   0   Birth asphyxia.
   0   Hypoglycaemia.

B +2 Chest X-ray.
   +2 Blood culture.
   +2 Fluoroscopy.
   +2 Ultrasound of diaphragm.

Maximum marks +8

The important points to note are: a history of prolonged rupture of membranes, maternal pyrexia. These are suggestive of infection, either pneumonia or septicaemia. The lowish pH and slightly elevated P_{CO_2} are further suggestive evidence of respiratory infection. However, a difficult delivery followed by an Erb's palsy are also suggestive of phrenic nerve involvement leading to tachypnoea.

Fluoroscopy or ultrasound of the diaphragm (real-time) are useful investigations if phrenic nerve palsy is suspected.

Question 17

A 6-year-old was referred by his General Practitioner because of a four-week history of episodic frontal headache associated with nausea and vomiting. The headaches lasted up to 1 hour and were not entirely relieved by simple analgesics. He also complained of 'light hurting his eyes'. The mother also said that he has lost weight over the past 8–9 months and had been nauseated with occasional small vomits.

Examination revealed a thin and lethargic boy. His temperature was 37°C, heart rate 70/min and blood pressure 110/65. There was no meningism and tendon reflexes were normal. Visualization of his fundi was not possible at the clinic because of extraneous light. There was no past-pointing. Romberg's sign was absent.

A   What is the most likely diagnosis?
B   What important step would you take next in the physical examinaton of this child?
C   Give two investigations which are most helpful in your management.

Answer to question 17

A +4 Raised intracranial pressure due to an intracranial tumour.
    +4 Intracranial tumour.
    0 Migraine.
    0 Meningitis.

B +2 Re-examination of the fundi in a darkened room after dilating the pupils.
    +2 Test the visual field.

C +2 CAT scan of the brain.
    +2 Skull X-ray to show mid-line shift.

Maximum marks +10

The fairly long history of persistent headaches and other symptoms, and weight loss are suggestive of an intracranial space-occupying lesion. Migraine attacks are episodic usually. There is nothing in the history or physical examination to suggest meningitis. The absence of any cerebellar signs does not rule out intracerebral tumours as one-third of intracranial tumours are supratentorial. These include the gliomas of the hemispheres, meningiomas and gliomas around the optic nerve and pituitary area. The medulloblastoma and astrocytoma are the commonest infratentorial tumours in childhood (accounting for about 75%).

    Beside causing symptoms like headache and vomiting which is due to raised intracranial pressure, supratentorial tumours may also impinge on the third nerve (dilating pupil), loss of visual field and drowsiness when the tumour impinges upon the brain stem. Infratentorial tumours are more likely to cause cerebellar symptoms like nystagmus and ataxia.

Question 18

An 18-month-old Caucasian girl was referred to the outpatient clinic with a history of irritability and pallor. Four weeks ago she had an episode of diarrhoea and vomiting. Since then she has not been feeding very well and continues to have occasional loose stools.

She is the only child of non-consanguinous parents. The father had an aortic valve replacement about 5 years ago and is on anticoagulant therapy. The mother is healthy but father's brother was said to have been treated for anaemia.

She was born at term. She was breast fed for 6 months and solids were introduced at 4 months. She sat up unaided at 7 months and walked at 13 months.

On examination she was not ill. Her height and weight were on the 25th percentile. The temperature was 37°C. Her heart rate was 100/min. There was no audible murmur. The spleen was palpable 2 cm below the costal margin and the liver was 2 cm below the costal margin. The rest of the physical examination was normal. Urinalysis showed no protein and no sugar.

Results of Investigations

HB 8.8 g/dl
WBC 5.8 × 10^9/l
    Normal differential count
Platelets 230 × 10^9/dl
Direct Coombs' test — negative

A   What is the most likely cause of the splenomegaly?
B   Give two investigations that would help in the diagnosis.

Answer to question 18

A +4 Congenital (hereditary) spherocytosis.
    +3 Congenital haemolytic anaemia (non-spherocytic).
    +1 Haemolytic anaemia.

B +2 Blood film.
    +2 Red cell fragility test.
    +2 Red cell enzyme studies.
    +2 Autohaemolysis test.

Maximum marks +8

Splenomegaly and anaemia in a Caucasian child, and a preceding history of infection are strongly suggestive of hereditary spherocytosis. The negative Coombs' test also suggests that the haemolytic anaemia is not auto-immune. Hereditary spherocytosis is an autosomal dominant condition and is more common among Europeans. Neonatal jaundice is present in about half of the patients. A crisis can be precipitated by any intercurrent infection. Splenomegaly is a constant finding but is not present in about 20% of cases.

As the defect is due to an abnormality of the red cell membrane, the red cell fragility test is diagnostic. Spherocytes can be easily seen in the blood film.

Other congenital haemolytic anaemias due to red cell enzyme deficiencies (e.g. pyruvate kinase, hexokinase etc.) usually show some spherocytes in the blood film, a positive autohaemolysis test but the Coombs' test is negative and Heinz bodies are absent. Specific diagnosis is by spectrophotometric enzyme assay of red cells. The autohaemolysis test measures the rate of spontaneous lysis of the patient's red cells when incubated at 37°C in their own plasma. It is positive in many types of congenital haemolytic anaemias.

Question 19

A 13-year-old boy was admitted to hospital following a road traffic accident in which he sustained a fracture of his left femur. He made good progress. However, on systematic enquiry, his mother complained that her son had not been growing very much over the past 2–3 years. He also had a dry scaly skin especially on his hands over the past 9 months. He felt tired easily and slept a lot. His teachers had remarked that he had 'lost the sparkle' in his personality. He was an only child of healthy parents. A cousin had asthma and eczema. The birth history was normal. He was bottle fed from birth. Other than mumps and chickenpox infection several years ago, he had been well. His developmental history was unremarkable.

On examination he was not ill. His weight was on the 75th percentile and his height was on the 10th percentile. He had dry scaly skin and some yellowish coloration of the skin of his hands and feet. His temperature was 37°C . The pulse rate was 80/min and his blood pressure was 98/50. The heart sounds were normal and there was no murmur. The muscle tone and power were normal. The knee jerks were equal and present. The ankle jerks showed slow relaxation. Both plantar responses were flexor. The examination of the respiratory and gastrointestinal systems was normal. Urinalysis showed no protein, blood or glucose.

Routine full blood count showed:

Haemoglobin 13.5 g/dl
WBC 8.4 × 10^9/l
Platelets 250 × 10^9/l

A What is the most likely diagnosis?
B Name three investigations that would be most helpful in this case.

Answer to question 19

A +4 Acquired hypothyroidism or juvenile hypothyroidism.
   +4 Autoimmune thyroiditis.
   +1 Obesity.
    0 Any muscular disorder.

B +2 Serum thyroxine level.
   +2 Serum thyroid stimulating hormone level.
   +2 Antithyroid antibodies.
   +2 Bone age.
   +2 Radioiodine uptake studies.
   +2 Electrocardiogram.
   +1 Serum cholesterol.

Maximum marks +10

The presence of myxoedematous skin, sluggish reflexes, growth delay and sleepiness in an obese child who has been previously well is strongly suggestive of acquired hypothyroidism. A goitre is not always present. Clinically it can be difficult to differentiate from autoimmune thyroiditis (Hashimoto's thyroiditis). In thyroiditis, some patients may have symptoms of hyperthyroidism instead. However, laboratory data in thyroiditis usually show the presence of antithyroid antibodies. Treatment is replacement with thyroxine.

Question 20

A 2-week-old girl was admitted to hospital as an emegency. She had been vomiting and not feeding for the past 36 hours. She is the third child of healthy parents. The birth history was normal and she was discharged home after 48 hours.

Examination revealed a dehydrated and ill child. The temperature was 36.6°C. Her heart rate was 160/min and BP 60/45. Her breath sounds were normal with equal air entry. The liver and spleen were not palpable. The labia were fused.

Initial blood tests showed:

HB 14.5 g/dl
WBC 9.5 × 10^9/l
Serum sodium 116 mmol/l
Serum potassium 6.2 mmol/l
Serum urea 10.5 mmol/l
Blood sugar 1.0 mmol/l

A What is the most likely diagnosis?
B What two urgent therapeutic measures would you take in this case?

Answer to question 20

A +4 Adrenocortical crisis due to congenital adrenal hyperplasia.
   +4 Congenital adrenal hyperplasia.
   +1 Hyponatraemic dehydration.

B +2 Intravenous fluids with normal saline and dextrose.
   +2 Intravenous hydrocortisone.
   +1 Intravenous fluids.
   +1 Face-mask oxygen.

Maximum marks +8

The presence of fused labia is an important sign in this case
although the nature of the clitoris was not mentioned. When this is
considered with the history of vomiting, dehydration and the serum
biochemistry results, a diagnosis of adrenocortical crisis due to
congenital adrenal hyperplasia ('salt-losing type') is most likely.
The replacement of fluid intravenously with normal saline and
dextrose is life-saving. Hydrocortisone should also be given.
Maintenance therapy will be required.

III Data interpretation

1 A 2-day-old term Chinese infant was noted to be jaundiced. Results of investigations are as follows:

Total serum bilirubin 250 μmol/l
Blood group A
Mother's blood group O
Direct Coombs' test negative

A What is the most likely diagnosis?
B Give one investigation that you would do to confirm the diagnosis.

2 A 4-month-old infant had a developmental assessment. The gross motor findings were as follows:

Head lag (45°) on traction
Lifts head above trunk level on ventral suspension
Unable to sit with tendency to fall backwards

What is the most likely problem with this infant?

3 A 3-week-old infant has not been feeding well. The urine chromatogram showed excess amount of valine, leucine and isoleucine.

What is the most likely diagnosis?

4 A 10-year-old child undergoes cardiac catheterization:

Results	Oxygen saturation (%)	Pressure (mm Hg)
SVC	70	—
RA	73	Mean 4
RV	83	48/3
PA	82	20/10
Femoral artery	88	84/55

What is the diagnosis?

Answers

1A +3 ABO incompatibility.
　　　+3 Glucose-6-phosphate dehydrogenase deficiency.
　　　+2 Congenital spherocytosis.
　　　0   Any haemoglobinopathy.

1B +2 Presence of IgG anti-A antibody in mother.
　　　+2 Assay red blood cell glucose-6-phosphate
　　　　　dehydrogenase activity.

Maximum marks +5

The blood group of mother and baby is ripe for an ABO
incompatibility set-up although the Coombs' test is negative.
It is positive in only 3% of cases with ABO incompatibility. As
the infant is Chinese, glucose-6-phosphate dehydrogenase
deficiency must be excluded. In this condition Coombs' test is
negative. Congenital spherocytosis is rare in the Chinese
people.

2 +4 Spastic cerebral palsy.
　　+1 Developmental delay.
　　0 Hypotonia.

Maximum marks +4

The excessive head lag and increased extensor tone are
suggestive of this condition. The presence of increased muscle
tone, knee jerks, sustained clonus and extensor plantars are
further confirmatory evidence.

3 +3 Maple syrup urine disease.
　　0 Any other answer.

Maximum marks +3

This condition is an inborn error of metabolism involving the
branch chain amino acids. It commonly presents in the first
week of life with feeding and respiratory problems. There are
often associated neurological symptoms like a shrill cry,
convulsion, spasticity leading to coma. The enzyme
abnormality (ketoacid decarboxylase) can be confirmed in the
white blood cell or cultured fibroblast enzyme assay.

4 +4 Small ventricular septal defect and pulmonary stenosis.
　　+2 Ventricular septal defect.
　　+2 Pulmonary stenosis.

Maximum marks +4

The results show an increase in oxygen saturation in the right
ventricle and a pressure gradient of 28 mm Hg across the
pulmonary valve which gives the diagnoses of ventricular
septal defect and pulmonary stenosis.

Questions

5   A 10-week-old boy presented with failure to thrive. He had
    been vomiting after each feed for the past 2 days. The initial
    investigations showed:

Serum sodium 132 mmol/l
Serum chloride 89 mmol/l
Serum potassium 3.0 mmol/l
Serum urea 6 mmol/l
Urine pH 6.1
Hb 13.5 g/dl
WBC 9.9×10^9/l

What is the most likely diagnosis?

6

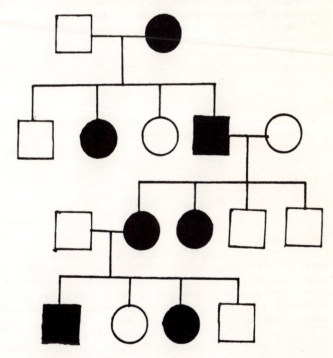

What is the mode of inheritance?

Answers

5   +3   Pyloric stenosis.
        +1   Intestinal obstruction.
        +1   Hyponatraemia.

Maximum marks +3

The history of failure to thrive, vomiting and decreased
serum sodium, potassium and chloride strongly suggest a
diagnosis of pyloric stenosis.

6   +3   X-linked dominant trait.
        +1   Autosomal dominant trait.

Maximum marks +3

Note that:
All daughters of affected men are affected.
No male-to-male transmission.
Half the daughters of affected women are affected.
Males more severely affected.

Questions

7

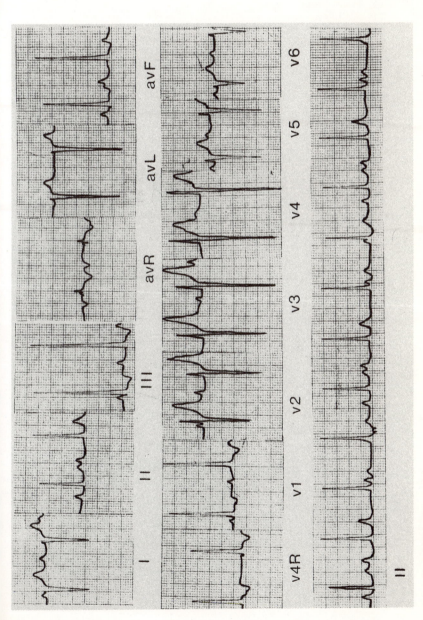

What is the abnormality?

Answers

7 +4   Complete AV or heart block.
   +2   Heart block.
   +2   AV block.
   0   AV dissociation.
   0   Ectopics.

Maximum marks +4

Any answer other than complete AV or heart block is not precise enough.

Questions

8 A 1-year-old boy was admitted to hospital with a history of vomiting. He was treated with antibiotics for a throat infection 3 days ago by his family doctor. On admission, his temperature was 39.5°C.

The results of the lumbar puncture were as follows:

Cell count:
240 polymorphs/mm^3
60 lymphocytes/mm^3
Protein concentration 0.8 g/l
Sugar concentration 2.8 mmol/l

A What is the most likely diagnosis?
B Give one further test which would be helpful in the diagnosis.

9 A 3-year-old girl had confirmed bacterial meningitis. Routine laboratory investigations showed these results:

Hb 10.5 g/dl
WBC 23 × 10^9/l
Blood sugar 5 mmol/l
Serum sodium 123 mmol/l
Potassium 3.5 mmol/l
Urea 1.8 mmol/l
Calcium 2.10 mmol/l

A What is the most likely explanation for the biochemical abnormalities?
B What important therapeutic measure would you take other than treatment with antibiotics?

Answers

8A   +3   Partially treated bacterial meningitis.
         +1   Viral meningitis.
         +1   Brain abscess.
         +1   Bacterial meningitis.

8B   +2   Counter-current electrophoresis on CSF.
         +2   Latex agglutination test on CSF.

Maximum marks +5

The somewhat mixed picture in the CSF findings and the history of previous antibiotic therapy should make one think of partially treated meningitis. Viral meningitis and brain abscess are the differential diagnosis although the somewhat short history would make the latter less likely.

Although the bacteria in the CSF may not be cultured, the polysaccharide cell wall may be detected by the methods listed.

9A   +3   Inappropriate antidiuretic hormone secretion.
         +1   Fluid overload.
         +1   Hyponatraemia.
          0   Hyponatraemic dehydration.

9B   +2   Fluid restriction.
          0   Correct hyponatraemia.

Maximum marks +5

The presence of low serum sodium in a patient with bacterial meningitis should make one think of probable inappropriate antidiuretic secretion. This should be confirmed by measuring the serum and urine osmolality. Fluid overload is a problem particularly with intravenous fluid infusion.

Management of inappropriate ADH secretion should be fluid restriction.

Questions

10 A 3-year-old girl who was born at 32 weeks' gestation had the following pure tone audiogram. The tympanogram curve and stapedius reflex were normal.

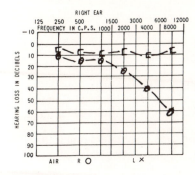
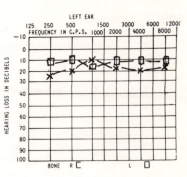

   A Report the audiogram.
   B What is the most likely cause?

11 A healthy child is able to build a tower of 4 cubes and aligns 3 cubes as a 'train' but unable to build a bridge or gate by imitation.

   What age would you put the motor skill of this child?

12 A 5-year-old boy had prolonged bleeding after tonsillectomy. The results of blood tests were as follows:

   Hb 10 g/dl
   WBC 8.5×10^9/l
   Platelet count 200×10^9/l
   PTT 65 s (control 43 s)
   PT 14 s (control 12 s)
   Bleeding time 5 minutes

   A What is the most likely diagnosis?
   B Give two tests that would confirm your diagnosis.

Answers

10A +2 Normal bone conduction bilaterally.
    +2 Normal hearing (for ordinary speech) but hearing loss on right for higher frequency.

10B +2 Hyperbilirubinaemia.
    +2 Idiopathic.
    +2 Congenital viral infections.

Maximum marks +6

The high-frequency hearing loss is typical of hyperbilirubinaemia. However, it is often bilateral. Congenital viral infections cannot be excluded. Not infrequently, no cause is found.
NB. With questions on audiograms, examiners prefer the term '. . . . . . hearing loss', rather than 'deafness'.

11 +4 2–2½ years.
    +1 3 years or 4 years.

Maximum marks +4

A 2-year-old is able to build a tower of at least 3 cubes. A 3-year-old is able to build a bridge by imitation and build a gate by 4 years.

12A +2 Classical haemophilia.
    +2 Christmas disease.
    +2 Von-Willebrand disease.

12B +2 Assay of factor VIII for haemophilia or assay of factor IX for Christmas disease.
    +2 Factor VIII antigen level.

Maximum marks +6

The prolonged PTT and normal platelet count are suggestive of a haemorrhagic disorder. As no family history was given, the diagnosis depends on specific factor assay. Factor VIII level may be low in von-Willebrand disease but the factor VIII antigen level is also reduced, unlike in haemophilia.

Questions

13 A 12-month-old child is referred by his general practitioner with a diagnosis of respiratory infection which has not responded to ampicillin and erythromycin despite 10 days of treatment. A full blood count showed:

Hb 12.4 g/dl
WBC 44 × 10^9/l
Neutrophil 28%
Lymphocytes 68%
Monocytes 3%
Eosinophils 1%
Film — moderate degree of toxic granulation

A What is the most likely diagnosis?
B Give an investigation that may confirm your diagnosis.

14 An 8-day-old, small for gestational age infant was noted to be losing weight despite taking an appropriate amount of milk. Results of investigations were as follows:

Serum sodium 150 mmol/l
Serum potassium 4.2 mmol/l
Serum urea 10.3 mmol/l
Blood sugar 21 mmol/l
Blood gases in room air
    pH 7.22
    Pco_2 4.3 kPa
    Po_2 9.3 kPa

What is the most likely diagnosis?

Answers

13A +3 Pertussis (or whooping cough).
   +2 Acute infectious lymphocytosis.
   +1 Viral infection.
   0   Pneumonia.

13B +2 *Bordetella pertussis* serology.
   +1 Pernasal swab for *B. pertussis* isolation.
   0   Blood culture.
   0   Chest X-ray.

Maximum marks +5

A white cell count of over 30 000 with over 60% lymphocytes is very suggestive of whooping cough. Acute infectious lymphocytosis is very similar but an eosinophilia is often present.

Serology to look for haemagglutinin or complement fixing (CF) antibodies. A pernasal swab for *Bordetella pertussis* is not useful because of prior erythromycin treatment. CF antibodies may be absent early in the disease but almost always present by the third week. Note that in infants under 6 months old, CF and haemagglutinin antibodies are often absent. Chest X-ray is usually normal unless there are complications. It is not a diagnostic test for pertussis.

14 +4 Neonatal diabetes mellitus.
   +1 Hypernatraemia.
   +1 Hypernatraemic dehydration.

Maximum marks +4

The grossly elevated blood sugar, dehydration, metabolic acidosis and history of weight loss are suggestive of neonatal diabetes mellitus. This is usually a transient condition but only time will determine whether the diabetic state is permanent. In the management, it is important to rehydrate the infant. Insulin is normally required but extreme care should be taken to avoid hypoglycaemia.

Questions

15 A 7-day-old Indian boy who has been bottle fed had a
generalized convulsion. Birth history was normal. Results of
initial laboratory investigations were as follows:

Serum sodium 135 mmol/l
Serum potassium 4.0 mmol/l
Serum calcium 1.45 mmol/l
Serum magnesium 0.6 mmol/l
Serum phosphate 2.7 mmol/l
Serum blood sugar 4 mmol/l

What is the most likely diagnosis?

16 A 7-year-old boy has been complaining of intermittent
headaches and vomiting. Routine laboratory investigations
showed these results:

Hb 8.6 g/dl
WBC 8.1 × 10^9/l
Serum sodium 135 mmol/l
Serum potassium 4.6 mmol/l
Serum calcium 1.75 mmol/l
Serum urea 32.5 mmol/l
Blood glucose 5.5 mmol/l
Urine contained a trace of protein and glucose

What is the most likely cause for this child's condition?

17 A 6-week-old infant has persistent jaundice. Investigations are
as follows:

Total serum bilirubin 200 μmol/l
Conjugated bilirubin 170 μmol/l
Serum alkaline phosphatase 320 iu/l
SGOT 147 iu/l
Prothrombin time 18 seconds, control 12 s
Partial thromboplastin time 42 seconds, control 35 s
Clinitest negative
Clinistix negative

A What is the most likely diagnosis?
B What two further tests would be most helpful to confirm
the diagnosis?

Answers

15 +4   Late neonatal tetany.
     +4   Neonatal hypoparathyroidism.
     +4   Late neonatal hypocalcaemia.
     +1   Hypocalcaemia.
     +1   Hypomagnaemia.

Maximum marks +4

The low serum calcium, elevated phosphate and marginally low magnesium level in a 1-week-old infant with a convulsion is suggestive of late neonatal tetany. This should be distinguished from early hypocalcaemia which occurs within the first 72 hours often associated with perinatal events, low birth weight or prematurity. Late neonatal tetany is often a form of transient hypoparathyroidism often associated with maternal vitamin D deficiency. Further useful investigations should include the serum biochemistry, including vitamin D level in the mother. Serum parathormone level will be low in the neonate.

16 +4   Chronic renal failure.
     +1   Uraemia.
     +1   Anaemia.

Maximum marks +4

The elevated serum urea, low calcium and anaemia are suggestive of chronic renal failure.

17A +3   Extrahepatic biliary atresia.
      +3   Neonatal hepatitis syndrome.
      +3   Alpha-1-antitrypsin deficiency.
      +3   Congenital viral infection (toxoplasmosis, rubella, cytomegalovirus or herpes).

17B +2   Liver biopsy for histology.
      +2   Alpha-1-antitrypsin level.
      +2 I^{131} rose bengal faecal excretion test.

Maximum marks +7

The picture is one of obstructive or conjugated hyperbilirubinaemia. Clinically it will be difficult to distinguish between the various causes.

The definitive diagnostic procedure is liver biopsy. Each of the listed conditions shows fairly typical histological features. I^{131} rose bengal faecal excretion test will show less than 5% excretion of the dye in 72 hours in cases of extrahepatic biliary atresia. A liver biopsy is still required for confirmation before laparotomy.

Questions

18 A 9-year-old girl had her lung function assessed using a Wright Peak Flow Meter.

The results during and after 10 minutes exercise are as follows:

Time after start of exercise (min)	PEFR (l/min)
0	250
3	255
6	255
10	250
15	210
20	160
25	130
30	180

A What abnormality is demonstrated?
B What is the most likely diagnosis?

19

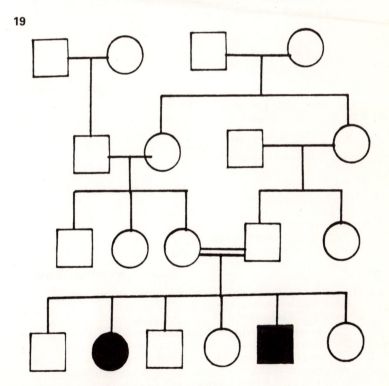

What is the mode of inheritance?

Answers

18A   +3   A reduction in PEFR following exercise due to bronchoconstriction.

18B   +2   Bronchial asthma.

Maximum marks +5

The PEFR clearly shows a slight rise on start of exercise followed by a decline after 10 minutes of exercise. This is characteristic of asthma. The PEFR should return to normal resting value later or it can be reversed by the use of a B_2-agonist.

19   +3   Autosomal recessive trait.
           +0   Any other answer.

Maximum marks +3

Note the horizontal transmission, consanguinous parents, both sexes are affected and in unaffected parents.

Questions

20

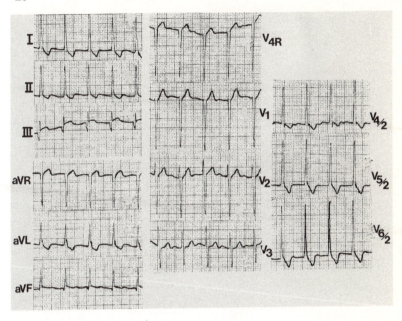

Give three abnormalities in this ECG.

21 A 5-day-old preterm infant had a lumbar puncture performed. The results are as follows:

White cell count   5 cells/mm³
Protein concentration   1.1 g/l
Glucose concentration   2.3 mmol/l
CSF/blood glucose (%)   85
Gram stain   No organism seen

What is the most likely diagnosis on the basis of these results?

Answers

20 +1 Gross left ventricular hypertrophy.
+1 Left ventricular strain.
+1 T-wave inversion in leads I, II, aVL, and left chest leads.
+1 Nodal rhythm.

Maximum marks +3

21 +4 Normal.
+1 Viral meningitis.
+1 Bacterial meningitis.

Maximum marks +4

Although meningitis can be present rarely in the presence of normal CSF findings, these results are within the norm for a preterm infant. (Reference: Sarff et al. Journal of Pediatrics 1976; 88: 473.)

Questions

22 A 6-year-old boy has a 1-week history of 'flu-like' illness and sore throat.
   Routine investigations show:

Hb 8.5 g/dl
WBC 8.5 × 10^9/l
Platelets 71 × 10^9/l
Serum sodium 131 mmol/l
Serum potassium 4.7 mmol/l
Serum creatinine 200 μmol/l
Blood sugar 4.5 mmol/l

What is the most likely diagnosis?

23 A 6-month-old boy presents with a history of poor feeding and slow weight gain. The following laboratory results were obtained:

Serum sodium 155 mmol/l
Serum potassium 5.5 mmol/l
Serum urea 12 mmol/l
Serum creatinine 90 μmol/l
   urine SG 1003
      pH 6.9
      protein negative
      glucose negative

What is the most likely condition that may cause this biochemical abnormality?

Answers

22 +4 Haemolytic uraemic syndrome.
+1 Acute glomerulonephritis.
+1 Anaemia.
+1 Uraemia.

Maximum marks +4

The finding of a low haemoglobin level, platelet count and elevated serum creatinine in a child with a history of antecedent infection is strongly suggestive of haemolytic uraemic syndrome. These features are typically preceded by a history of gastroenteritis or a 'flu-like' illness. Acute renal failure due to acute glomerulonephritis may give a similar picture but one would not expect a low Hb or platelet count.

23 +4 Nephrogenic diabetes insipidus.
+2 Overconcentrated feeds.
+2 Hypernatraemia.
0   Dehydration.

Maximum marks +4

The presence of a very dilute urine despite the presence of dehydration, elevated sodium concentration and abnormal renal function are suggestive of nephrogenic diabetes insipidus. The rather dilute urine makes the diagnoses of overconcentrated feeds and hypernatraemia less likely.

Questions

24 An 18-day-old Asian boy who is bottle fed had two episodes of
cyanosis and twitching. Results of investigations are as
follows:

Hb 14.2 g/dl
WBC 12 × 10⁹/l
Serum calcium 2.02 mmol/l
SGOT 93 iu/l
Alkaline phosphatase 300 iu/l
Triglyceride 9.5 mmol/l (NR less than 1.9)
Uric acid 538 μmol/l (NR 120–360)
Lactate 7.5 mmol/l (NR less than 1.4)
Postprandial (1 hour) blood sugar 3.6 mmol/l
Preprandial blood sugar 0.5 mmol/l

A What is the most likely diagnosis?
B What two tests would you do to confirm the diagnosis?

25

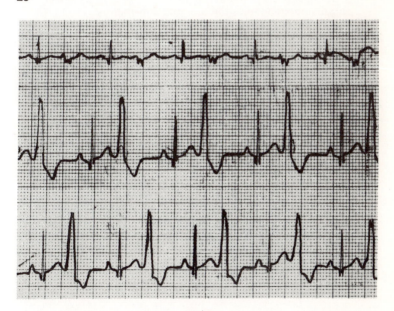

A What abnormality is shown in this ECG?
B What is the most likely cause?

Answers

24A +3 Glycogen storage disease, type I or III.
+2 Glycogen storage disorder.
+1 Hypoglycaemia.

24B +2 Liver biopsy to assay Glucose-6-phosphatase or amylo-l-6-glucosidase.
+2 RBC or leucocyte glucose-6-phosphatase or amylo-l-6-glucosidase activity.
+1 Glucagon test.
+1 Galactose load test.

Maximum marks +7

Convulsion, fasting hypoglycaemia, hyperlipidaemic, lactate acidosis and elevated uric acid level are strongly suggestive of glycogen storage disease type I (von Gierke) or III (Cori). Hepatomegaly and short stature are further features.

A liver biopsy to assay the specific enzyme activity or RBC or leucocyte enzyme assay will confirm the diagnosis.

Both the glucagon and the galactose loading tests will suggest the diagnosis but are not confirmatory.

25A +3 Ventricular bigeminy.
+1 Coupled beats.
+1 Fixed ventricular premature beat.
0 Ectopics.

25B +2 Digoxin.

Maximum marks +5

The rhythm alternates between a regular sinus beat and a ventricular premature beat. There is usually a constant interval between the sinus beat and the ventricular premature beat, i.e. fixed coupling, indicating that by some means the sinus beat controls the discharge of the ventricular ectopic focus. Digoxin is a common cause of ventricular premature contractions and characteristically produces ventricular bigeminy.

Questions

26 A 3-year-old Pakistani child who had no previous history of convulsions was admitted with status epilepticus. Results of initial investigations showed:

Hb 6.5 g/dl
WBC 6.8 × 10⁹/l
Blood sugar 5.5 mmol/l
Serum sodium 135 mmol/l
Serum potassium 4.0 mmol/l
Serum urea 6.0 mmol/l
CSF opening pressure 23 cm H$_2$O
CSF cell count less than 10 WBC
CSF protein 1.8 g/l
CSF sugar 4 mmol/l
Urine protein +++ blood +
Clinitest 1%

A What is the most likely diagnosis?
B Give an investigation to confirm your diagnosis.

27 A 14-month-old Pakistani boy attended outpatient clinic because of 'poor appetite'. A full blood count was sent by his family doctor. The results were:

Hb 5.8 g/dl
WBC 5 × 10⁹/l
(60% lymphocytes, 36% neutrophils, 3% monocytes, 1% eosinophils)
MCV 54 fl
MCH 18 pg
MCHC 32 g/l
Platelets 200 × 10⁹/dl
Blood film shows target cells and polychromasia

A What is the likely diagnosis?
B Give three further investigations that would be most helpful.

Answers

26A +4 Lead encephalopathy.
      0   Meningitis.

26B +2 Serum lead level.
      +2 X-ray of long bones.
      +2 Look for basophilic stippling in white blood cells.

Maximum marks +6

The presence of anaemia, increased intracranial pressure, raised CSF protein and evidence of tubular damage are suggestive of this condition. There is no suggestion of bacterial or viral meningitis. The diagnosis can be confirmed by measuring the serum lead level. The basophils may show stippling. Lead lines may be seen in the epiphysis of long bones.

27A +2 Iron deficiency anaemia.
      +2 B-thalassaemia major.
      +2 B-thalassaemia trait with iron deficiency anaemia.
      +2 B-thalassaemia trait.

27B +2 Serum iron and iron binding capacity.
      +2 Serum ferritin level.
      +2 Haemoglobin electrophoresis.
      +2 HbF and A_2 estimation.
      +2 Haematological tests on parents.

Maximum marks +8

It is not possible to make a definitive diagnosis on the basis of the given blood test results. It shows a microcytic, hypochromic anaemia. The presence of target cells and polychromasia are common to many haemoglobinopathies. Further tests like those listed are required to confirm the diagnosis.

Questions

28   A milk preparation when reconstituted has the following constituents per 100 ml:

Protein 3.9 g
Fat 3.2 g
Carbohydrate 4.6 g
Sodium 33 mg
Potassium 60 mg
Calcium 120 mg
Phosphate 44 mg

Give two reasons why this milk is unsuitable for a 1-month-old baby.

29   A 3-year-old boy has the following pure-tone audiogram. The tympanogram curve was flat but the stapedius reflex was normal on both ears.

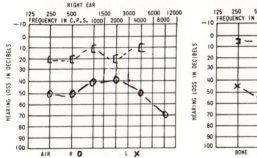
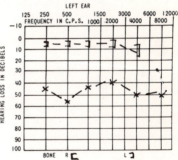

A   What is the abnormality?
B   What is the underlying cause?

Answers

28 +2 Protein content is too high.
+2 Calcium content is too high.

Maximum marks +4

Artificial formula milk feeds should contain no more than 1.9 g protein per 100 ml. Calcium content should be in the region of 40–50 mg per 100 ml.

29A +2 Bilateral moderate conductive hearing loss.

29B +2 Glue ears.

Maximum marks +4

A flat tympanogram with normal stapedius reflex is suggestive of glue ears.

Questions

30 This is the karyotype of a neonate.

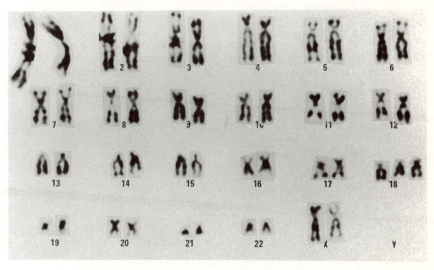

A How would you designate this karyotype?
B Name three major clinical features that may be found in this baby.

Answers

30A +3 Trisomy 18.
         +2 Edward's syndrome.

30B +1 These include congenital heart disease (VSD, PDA),
             micronagthia, low-set malformed ears, low birth weight,
             flexion deformity of fingers, rockerbottom feet,
             equinovarus, cleft lip ± palate, hypoplasia of fingernails,
             webbed neck, mental retardation, failure to thrive.

Maximum marks +6

The answer Edward's syndrome scores less marks because the
question asks for the karyotype.

IV Projected material

Question 1

A 7-year-old child is admitted acutely ill. What is the most likely diagnosis?

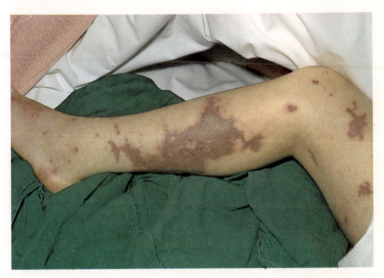

Answer to question 1

+4   Meningococcal septicaemia.
+1   Septicaemia due to other organisms.
0   Leukaemia.
0   Purpura.

Maximum marks +4

The rash of acute meningococcaemia may arise within hours of onset of infection. The rash can be morbilliform, petechial or purpuric. Severe and extensive purpuric lesions may later slough off leaving deep skin lesions.

Question 2

An 11-month-old infant is referred by his family doctor.

A What is the diagnosis?
B Give two likely causes.

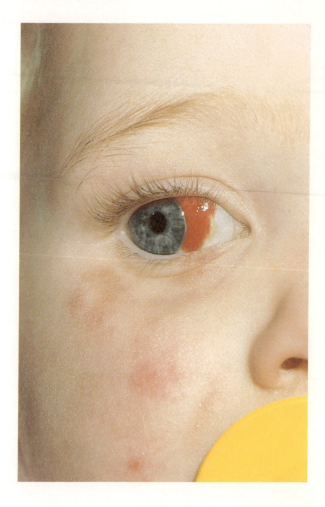

Answer to question 2

A +2 Subconjunctival haemorrhage.
B +2 Trauma.
  +2 Trauma due to non-accidental injury.
  +2 Whooping cough.
  +2 Excessive straining.

Maximum marks +6

Subconjunctival haemorrhage may appear like episcleritis and scleritis, but unlike these conditions it does not obscure the vascular layer. No treatment is normally required.

Question 3

This is the repeat cranial ultrasound scan of an infant at 2 weeks old. What is the most important abnormality shown in this scan?

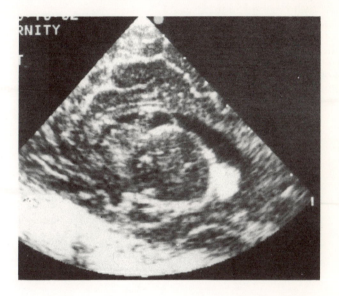

Answer to question 3

+3   Resolving intraventricular blood clot over the germinal
      area.
+1   Intraventricular haemorrhage.

Maximum marks +3

The cranial ultrasound clearly shows the resolving blood clot.
The dense area in the posterior horn is part of the choroid
plexus. Intraventricular haemorrhage becomes less likely after 2
weeks of age.

Question 4

This child is $2\frac{1}{2}$ years old. What is the most likely diagnosis?

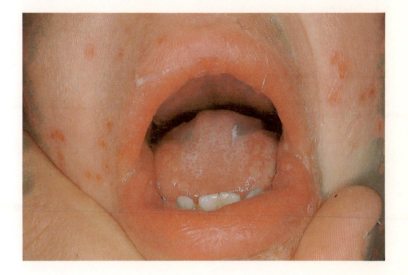

Answer to question 4

+3   Herpes simplex gingivostomatitis (or infection).
+1   Mouth ulcers.
0   Oral thrush.

Maximum marks +3

This picture is typical of primary herpes simplex infection. Note the crops of ulceration in the mouth, mucous membranes, lips and around the mouth.

Question 5

This is a Gram stain of the CSF of a 2-year-old child. What is the diagnosis?

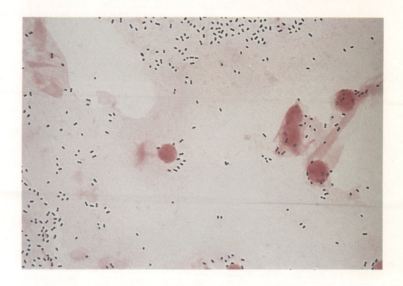

Answer to question 5

+4   *Streptococcus pneumoniae* meningitis.
+3   Bacterial meningitis of any sort.
+1   Meningitis.

Maximum marks +4

The picture shows numerous Gram positive diplococci.
Haemophilus influenza and *N. meningitidis* are Gram-negative
organisms (stain red with Gram's stain).

Question 6

This is a neonate. What is the most likely diagnosis?

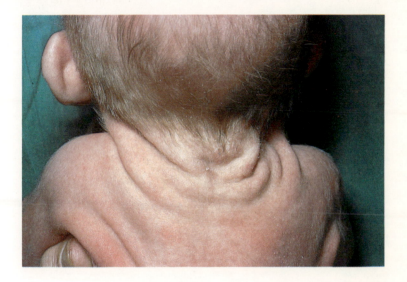

Answer to question 6

+3   Turner's syndrome.

Maximum marks +3

The picture shows loose skin folds at the nape of the low
hairline. These are fairly typical of Turner's syndrome.
Diagnosis should be confirmed by chromosomal analysis.

Question 7

This is a neonate. What is the most likely diagnosis?

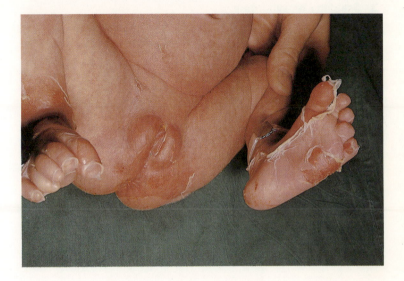

Answer to question 7

+3   Toxic epidermal necrolysis.
+3   Lyell's disease.
+3   Scalded skin syndrome.

Maximum marks +3

This is often due to a staphylococcal skin infection but it could be a hypersensitivity phenomenon triggered by many factors including drugs. The child develops fever, malaise, a generalized rash with localized skin tenderness and erythema. Gentle pressure on the skin will denude it (Nikolsky's sign). Bullae formation may occur followed by desquamation. Systemic antibiotic is indicated.

Question 8

A   This infant is born to healthy Pakistani parents. What is the
    lesion shown?
B   What treatment is required?

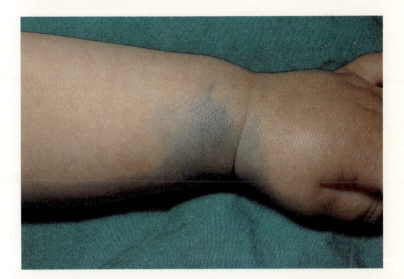

Answer to question 8

A   +3   Mongolian blue spot.
    +1   Pigmented naevus.
B   +2   No treatment.

Maximum marks +5

Mongolian blue spots are usually greyish. They occur in some 80% of the Asiatic and black race and in about 10% of white infants. They usually occur over the presacral or low lumbar region but are present on shoulders and limbs. They may fade somewhat in the toddler years but can be present up to 9–10 years of age. No treatment is required.

Question 9

A child is admitted to hospital for investigations. What is the main feature shown in this slide?

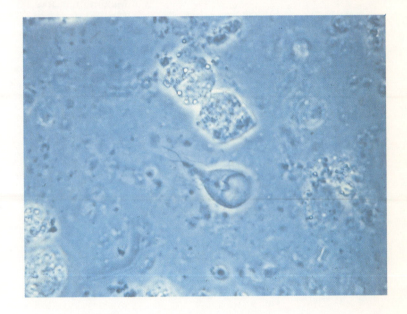

Answer to question 9

+3   Giardia lamblia.
0   Any other answer.

Maximum marks +3

The picture clearly shows the protozoa with its characteristic oval-shaped body with its flagella. Giardiasis may cause prolonged diarrhoea and failure to thrive. Treatment is with a course of metronidazole.

Question 10

This child was referred to hospital by his family doctor because of
pallor and abdominal pain.

A What is the procedure?
B What does it show?

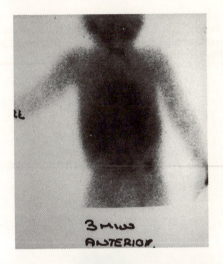

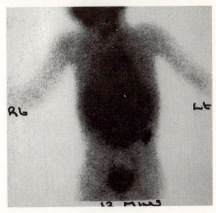

Answer to question 10

A +3 Technetium isotope scan.
  +1 Isotope scan.
B +2 'Hot-spot' (Meckel's diverticulum) over the left iliac fossa.

Maximum marks +5

The technetium is taken up by gastric mucosa and any other structure containing gastric mucosa. In this case, a 'hot-spot' is shown in the left iliac fossa.

Question 11

This infant required resuscitation at birth. What is the radiological abnormality?

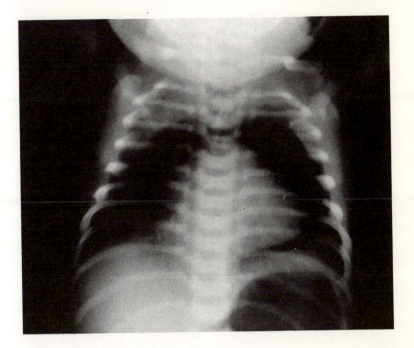

Answer to question 11

+4   Pneumomediastinum.
0   Bilateral pneumothorax.
0   Pneumopericardium.

Maximum marks +4

This is a pneumomediastinum because the air is essentially central with some of it overlying the left heart border. It is not a pneumothorax because lung fields can be seen to the edge. In pneumopericardium the upper border of the air will be limited by the root of the heart.

Question 12

This is a female term infant. What is the diagnosis?

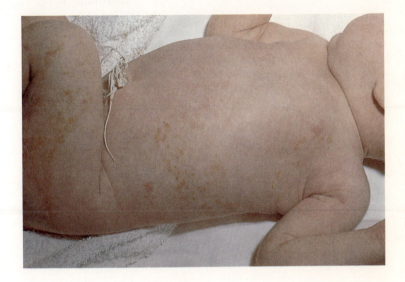

Answer to question 12

+3   Incontinentia pigmenti.

Maximum marks +3

This is an X-linked dominant condition. Within a few days of birth, there is a widespread vesicular eruption followed by warty papules over previous lesions. The lesions involute and become hyperpigmented producing typical streaky or whorled pattern.

Question 13

This 6-year-old girl complains of tiredness and anorexia. What is the most likely diagnosis?

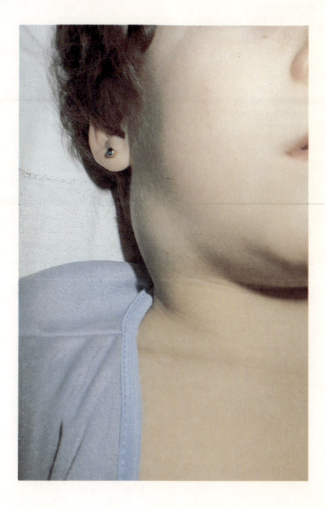

Answer to question 13

+3 Glandular fever or infectious mononucleosis.
+3 Cervical abscess.
+3 Lymphoma.
+3 Cervical lymphadenitis.
+1 Mumps.

Maximum marks +3

The picture shows a cervical swelling which is most likely to be
lymph nodes. The swelling in mumps is the parotid gland
which is higher.

Question 14

This child complains of spots over his abdomen only. What is the most likely diagnosis?

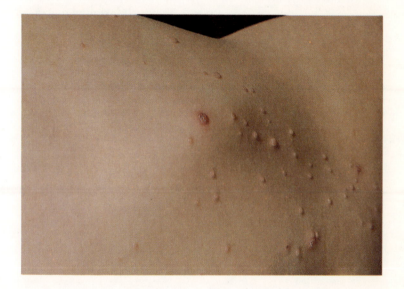

Answer to question 14

+3   Molluscum contangiosum.
+1   Warts.
+1   Chickenpox.

Maximum marks +3

The picture shows a crop of pearly papular lesions, one of
which appears infected. These are typical lesions of molluscum
contangiosum which is caused by a pox virus. The papule has a
characteristic central punctum. Treatment is by phenolization,
cryotherapy or curretage. Many will resolve spontaneously.

Question 15

This is the bone marrow smear of an infant who has slow development and hepatosplenomegaly.

A   What is the main feature shown?
B   What is the most likely diagnosis?

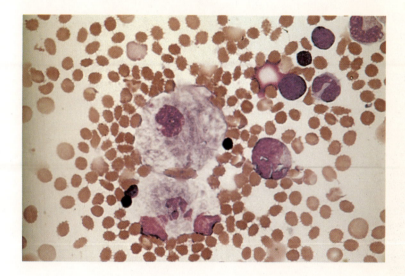

Answer to question 15

A +2 Gaucher's cell.
   +2 Foamy cell.
   0   Any other answer.
B +3 Gaucher's disease.
   +3 Niemann–Pick disease.
   0   Glycogen storage disease.

Maximum marks +5

The picture shows a typical Gaucher's cell with the blue-staining cytoplasm with a 'crinkled-silk' appearance. In Niemann–Pick disease the cell has a characteristic foamy appearance instead.

Question 16

This 6-year-old girl complains of general malaise and weight loss. What is the most likely diagnosis?

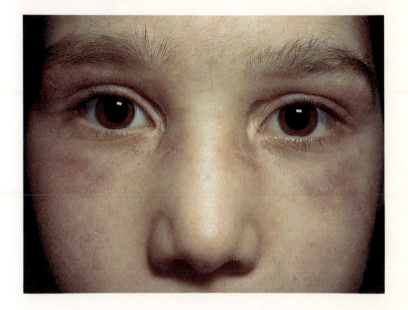

Answer to question 16

+4   Dermatomyositis.
+1   Systemic lupus erythematosus.

Maximum marks +5

The picture shows the typical violaceous heliotrope rash in the periorbital region which is consistent with a diagnosis of dermatomyositis. In systemic lupus erythematosus, the rash extends from the malar region to the bridge of the nose in a butterfly distribution.

Question 17

This is a neonate.

A What is the most likely diagnosis?
B What is the treatment?

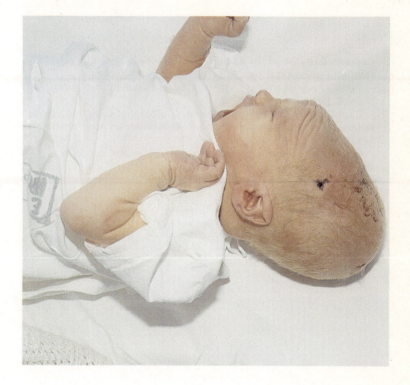

Answer to question 17

A   +3   Cephalhaematoma.
    +3   Caput succedaneum.
B   +2   No treatment required.
    +2   None. Reassure parents.

Maximum marks +5

Caput is oedema of the scalp caused by the presenting part of the head pressing through the partially dilating cervix.

Cephalhaematoma is swelling due to a collection of blood in the sub-pericranium.

Caput, unlike cephalhaematoma, characteristically lies across suture lines and it pits on pressure. It is maximal after birth and resolves within a few days.

Cephalhaematoma normally grows in size and can take months to resolve.

Question 18

This boy is admitted to hospital acutely ill. What is the diagnosis?

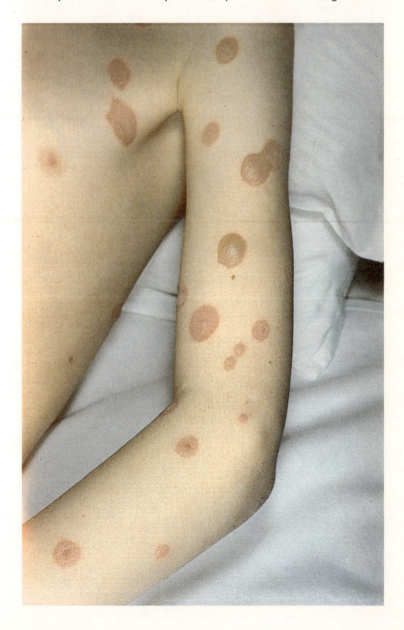

Answer to question 18

+4   Stevens–Johnson syndrome.
+3   Erythema multiforme.
+1   Drug eruption.
+1   Bullous urticaria.

Maximum marks +4

Stevens–Johnson syndrome is the severe form of erythema multiforme. It involves the mucous membranes in especially the mouth and eyes. The patient is also toxic. Systemic steroid is often used in the treatment. Mild erythema multiforme is characterized by target lesions. It remits spontaneously.

Question 19

What is the most likely diagnosis?

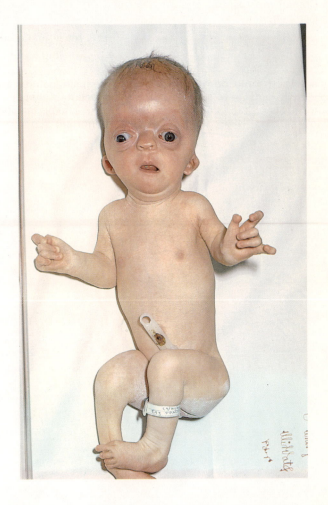

Answer to question 19

+4   Crouzon's disease.
+2   Craniosynostosis.
+1   Acrocephaly.

Maximum marks +4

This is an autosomal dominant condition. The main features are acrocephaly (closure of coronal suture), prominent forehead, proptosis, beak-shaped nose, hypoplastic maxilla, hypertension and low-set ears. Their intelligence is usually normal.

Question 20

This is the X-ray of long bones of a 14-month-old infant.

A Give two radiological abnormalities.
B What is the most likely diagnosis?

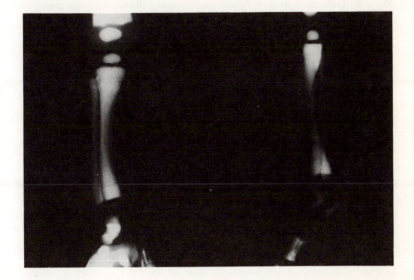

Answer to question 20

A +2 Increased density of bones.
    +2 Clubbing of metaphyses.
    +2 Irregular modelling of bone.
    +2 Lack of trabecular pattern.
B +2 Osteopetrosis or Albers–Schönberg disease or marble-bone disease.

Maximum marks +6

This condition can occur in the severe or mild form. The basic pathogenesis is not fully understood. There is a persistent calcification of the cartilaginous matrix. The bone is poorly modelled with no cortical definition. The entire bony structure is sclerotic and fragile. Haemopoeisis is also impaired.

V Multiple choice questions

SECTION A

A 2-year-old child is brought to hospital following acute ingestion of an unkown amount of aspirin. Recognized findings include:

1. Respiratory alkalosis.
2. Metabolic alkalosis.
3. A prolonged prothrombin time.
4. Pyrexia
5. Hypoglycaemia.

In toddlers' diarrhoea:

6. There is a proven association with cows' milk protein intolerance.
7. Failure to thrive is a recognized presenting feature.
8. A lactose-free diet is the treatment of choice.
9. There is a recognized association with atopy in children.
10. The jejunal biopsy shows mild villous atrophy.

Inguinal hernia in an infant:

11. Is differentiated from hydrocoele by the lack of definition of its upper pole on palpation.
12. Typically resolve spontaneously by 1 year of age.
13. Is more common in pre-term infants than term infants.
14. Is often associated with a hydrocoele.
15. Is very rarely complicated by strangulation.

Recognized clinical features of cardiac failure in infants include:

16. Pulsus paradoxus.
17. Splenomegaly.
18. Sweating.
19. Poor weight gain.
20. Flaring of the alae nasi.

Answers

1 **True** — salicylates stimulate the respiratory centre leading to an increase in the depth and rate of respiration. Carbon dioxide is eliminated and respiratory alkalosis results.

2 **False** — lactates accumulate leading to metabolic acidosis.

3 **True** — this is probably due to defective synthesis of clotting factors in the liver.

4 **True.**

5 **True.**

6 **False.**

7 **False** — patients are usually well and thriving.

8 **False** — there is no good evidence of lactose intolerance.

9 **False.**

10 **False** — the jejunal histology is usually normal.

11 **True.**

12 **False** — hydrocoele, rather than inguinal hernia may resolve.

13 **True.**

14 **True.**

15 **False** — strangulation is the most important complication and is not uncommon.

16 **False** — pulsus alternans is a characteristic sign of heart failure, not pulsus paradoxus. Pulsus alternans is a characteristic finding of left-sided heart failure.

17 **True** — the spleen may enlarge in association with venous congestion. Hepatomegaly is commoner.

18 **True.**

19 **True.**

20 **True** — tachypnoea is a common feature.

Questions

The following statements are true of opiate withdrawal in a newborn infant:

21 Naloxone should be given soon after birth to lessen any withdrawal symptoms.
22 Excessive yawning is a recognized feature.
23 Excessive sneezing is a recognized feature.
24 The Moro reflex is commonly absent.
25 Chlorpromazine is an effective drug for treating the symptoms.

The Juvenile Court in the United Kingdom:

26 Deals only with offences committed by children aged between 10–17 years old.
27 When in session, is closed to the public.
28 Has the power to sentence a juvenile to a detention centre.
29 When in session, is chaired by a judge.
30 Is the appropriate body to which to apply for a place of safety order.

Mental retardation is a usual finding in:

31 Prader–Willi syndrome.
32 Glycogen storage disease type I.
33 Alkaptonuria.
34 Galactosaemia.
35 Klinefelter's syndrome.

Answers

21 **False** — naloxone an opiate antagonist, is contraindicated in the management of neonatal opiate withdrawal. It may cause acute withdrawal symptoms which may be fatal.

22 **True.**

23 **True** — the neonate exhibits many features of central and autonomic nervous system dysfunction. Other features include restlessness, excessive wakefulness, high-pitched cry, tremors, hypertonicity and Moro reflexes, convulsions, hyperthermia, vomiting, diarrhoea, sweating, nasal snuffles, tachycardia, hypertension.

24 **False.**

25 **True** — diazepam, phenobarbitone and tincture of opium are also used.

26 **True** — offences committed by children aged 10–13 years and young persons (14–17 years) are under the jurisdiction of the Juvenile Court.

27 **True** — furthermore the names of the children appearing cannot be disclosed to the public.

28 **True** — the sentences given by the Juvenile Court include absolute discharge; conditional discharge; fine; supervision order; care order; and attendance centre order. With very young persons, in addition to above, they can also be sentenced to a detention centre.

29 **False** — there are three magistrates who are lay people and they are aided by the court clerk who is a professional solicitor or barrister.

30 **False** — any person can apply to a magistrate at any time for a place of safety order which is effective for up to 28 days.

31 **True** — a syndrome of hypotonia, hypogonadism, hypomentia and obesity with tendency to diabetes mellitus deficiency of glucose-6-phosphatase, large liver.

32 **False** — normal IQ unless having frequent severe hypoglycaemic attacks.

33 **False** — defect of tyrosine metabolism leading to accumulation of homogentisic acid. Stains cartilage and tissues. Asymptomatic.

34 **False** — deficiency of galactokinase. Normal intellect. Risk of cataracts.

35 **False** — mental retardation is rare. If present, is usually mild and may not be much more frequent than in the general population.

Questions

In coeliac disease:

36 The characteristic blood picture is of a microcytic anaemia.
37 Serum red cell folate is elevated.
38 The management includes a diet low in gluten.
39 The diet can be relaxed after 5 years treatment.
40 The histological appearance of the jejunal biopsy can be mimicked in cows' milk protein intolerance.

The following statements are recognized features of an innocent murmur:

41 The murmur is pansystolic.
42 The murmur commonly extends into diastole.
43 The intensity of the murmur varies with posture.
44 The murmur radiates commonly to the back.
45 The murmur is due to a small ventricular septal defect.

A simple febrile convulsion:

46 Occurs in the majority of infants less than 6 months old.
47 Usually lasts less than 15 minutes.
48 If it occurs more than twice in a year is an indication for long-term anti-convulsants.
49 If recurrent, is associated with an increased risk of intellectual deficit.
50 Is associated with a characteristic EEG 3/sec spike-wave pattern.

Recognized presenting features of acute lymphoblastic leukaemia of childhood include:

51 Fever.
52 Nocturia.
53 Bone pains.
54 Failure to thrive.
55 Haemarthrosis.

The following statements are correct:

56 A low birth weight infant is one of 2000 g and less.
57 A preterm infant is one of less than 37 completed weeks gestation.
58 A small for gestational age infant is one of less than 2000 g at 37 weeks' gestation.
59 The perinatal mortality rate refers to the number of deaths per 1000 live births per annum.
60 The early neonatal mortality rate refers to deaths in the first week of life per 1000 births.

Answers

36 True — microcytic anaemia of iron deficiency is typical.
37 False — it is usually low.
38 False — the diet must be totally gluten-free.
39 False — life-long adherence to a gluten-free regime is
          necessary.
40 True.

41 False.
42 False.
43 True.
44 False.
45 False.

46 False — it occurs between the age of 6 months to 7 years and
          is most frequent in the second year of life.
47 True — it usually lasts less than 15 minutes.
48 False.
49 False.
50 False.
51 True.
52 False.
53 True.
54 False — acute lymphoblastic leukaemia is more acute. There
          is no time for failure to thrive.
55 False — bruises rather than haemarthrosis (in haemophilia)
          are common features.

56 False — less than 2500 g.
57 True.
58 False — small for gestational age refers to infants whose birth
          weights are less than 10th percentile for age.
59 False — perinatal mortality rate refers to deaths per 1000 *live*
          and *still*birth.
60 False — early neonatal mortality rate refers to deaths per
          1000 *live* births only.

Questions

Recognized features of Fallot's tetralogy include:

61 Finger clubbing.
62 A loud second heart sound.
63 A pansystolic murmur.
64 A metabolic alkalosis.
65 A 'boot-shape' heart on chest radiograph.

A normal 2-year-old is able to do the following:

66 Walk on tiptoes when asked.
67 Copies a cross.
68 Build a tower of 9 bricks.
69 Know 3 parts of his body.
70 Name 3 colours.

In juvenile chronic arthritis:

71 Uveitis is a recognized complication.
72 The serum immunoglobulin level is raised.
73 The test for rheumatoid factor is positive in 50% of patients with multiple joint involvement.
74 The knee is rarely affected.
75 Soluble aspirin is of little value under the age of 5 in the treatment of children.

The following statements are correct:

76 One fluid ounce is about 30 ml.
77 The blood volume of a 3 kg newborn infant is about 450 ml.
78 The average caloric requirement of a 1 month old infant is about 100 kcal/kg/day
79 Cows' milk contains more protein per 100 ml than human milk.
80 Standard cows' milk formulae baby milks contain an average of 100 kcal/100 ml.

Recognized features of β-thalassaemia trait include:

81 A microcytic anaemia.
82 Gross hepatosplenomegaly.
83 Failure to thrive.
84 Low serum iron.
85 Raised HbA_2.

Answers

61 **True.**
62 **False.**
63 **True.**
64 **False**
65 **True.**

66 **False** — can walk tiptoes by $2\frac{1}{2}$–3 years.
67 **False** — can copy a cross by 3 years. Able to copy a diamond at 5 years.
68 **False** — can build a tower of 9 bricks by 3 years.
69 **True.**
70 **False.**

71 **True.**
72 **True** — any or all of the serum immunoglobulins may be raised.
73 **False** — rheumatoid factor is positive in only 10% of polyarticular juvenile chronic arthritis.
74 **False** — any synovial joint may be affected. Large joints, knees, elbows, ankles and wrists are commonly affected first.
75 **False.**

76 **True.**
77 **False** — the blood volume of a term infant is about 85 ml/kg.
78 **True.**
79 **True** — cows' milk contains about three times more protein.
80 **False** — it contains an average of 67 kcal/100 ml.

81 **True** — the red cells are microcytic and hypochromic with poikilocytosis.
82 **False** — hepatosplenomegaly is a feature in thalassaemia major because of increased extramedullary haematopoiesis and also haemasiderosis.
83 **False** — growth is normal in contrast to thalassaemia major.
84 **False** — serum iron level is normal or slightly raised.
85 **True** — about 90% of patients have raised HbA_2 of 3.4–7.0%.

Questions

The Moro reflex

86 Is present only in infants greater than 37 weeks' gestation.
87 Cannot be elicited after 6 months in normal infants.
88 Is not affected by sedation.
89 Is decreased in hypertonic infants.
90 Is absent in a young infant developing cerebral palsy.

Threadworm (*Enterobius vermicularis*) infection:

91 Is a recognized cause of acute abdominal pain in a young child.
92 Is a cause of generalized pruritus at night.
93 Is known to cause steatorrhoea.
94 Is best treated with mepacrine.
95 Results in intense eosinophilia in peripheral blood.

Recognized features of acute iron poisoning include:

96   Melaena.
97   Metabolic alkalosis.
98   Haemoglobinuria.
99   Hypotension.
100 Constipation.

Answers

86 **False** — it is nearly always present in preterm infants except the very low birth weight infants.

87 **True** — it disappears by 4 months and cannot be elicited by 6 months.

88 **False** — it is decreased or absent if the infant or mother has been heavily sedated.

89 **True** — this is due to inhibition of movements by the increased muscle tone.

90 **False** — the Moro reflex tends to persist longer than 6 months.

91 **False** — threadworm infection usually do not cause symptoms except perianal itching.

92 **False.**

93 **False.**

94 **False** — piperazine is the drug of choice and the whole family may need treatment.

95 **False** — eosinophilia is not seen because there is no tissue invasion.

96 **True.**

97 **False.**

98 **False.**

99 **True.**

100 **False.**

Questions

SECTION B

In Henoch–Schönlein purpura:

1 The bleeding time is prolonged.
2 Polyuria is an early sign of renal involvement.
3 Severe abdominal pain can respond to steroid therapy.
4 Intussusception is a recognized complication.
5 Total bedrest is recommended until skin lesions have disappeared.

Bronchiolitis:

6 Is characterized by an inspiratory wheeze and fine crackles through both lung fields.
7 Can be treated effectively with nebulized salbutamol.
8 If severe, frequently responds to intravenous steroid treatment.
9 Causes marked lymphopenia in the peripheral blood film.
10 May cause an inappropriate secretion of antidiuretic hormone.

The following vaccines contain live (or live attenuated) organisms:

11 Measles.
12 Rubella.
13 Poliomyelitis (Salk).
14 Cholera.
15 Hepatitis B.

Recognized features of acute idiopathic thrombocytopenia are:

16 Prolonged prothrombin time.
17 Antecedent infection.
18 Moderate splenomegaly.
19 Anaemia.
20 Leucopenia.

Presenting features of a child with hearing problems include:

21 Stammer.
22 Learning difficulties.
23 Enuresis.
24 Delayed motor development.
25 Behaviour problems.

Answers

1 **False** — bleeding time remains normal.
2 **False** — polyuria is not a feature.
3 **True.**
4 **True.**
5 **False** — bedrest makes no difference to the resolution of the condition.

6 **False** — expiratory wheezing is characteristic of small airway obstruction. Fine rales are heard at the end of inspiration and during early expiration.
7 **False.**
8 **False** — there is no proved evidence that salbutamol or steroids are of any help.
9 **False** — the differential white blood cell is usually normal.
10 **True** — this is an uncommon but recognized finding.

11 **True.**
12 **True.**
13 **False** — the Sabin vaccine contains live virus.
14 **False.**
15 **False.**

16 **False** — the clotting studies are usually normal.
17 **True** — in about 70% of cases, there is a history of infection.
18 **False** — the spleen is not normally enlarged in ITP. Significant splenomegaly should make one question the diagnosis.
19 **False** — anaemia is not a feature unless there is significant blood loss.
20 **False** — the white cell count and morphology are normal.

21 **False.**
22 **True** — this should always alert the clinician to possible hearing defects.
23 **False.**
24 **False.**
25 **True** — children with major hearing loss also have short attention spans.

Questions

Undescended testis:

26 Usually descend spontaneously after the first year of life.
27 Should be treated by orchidopexy between 4 and 6 years of age.
28 Should be treated with hormones prior to surgery in all cases.
29 Is known to be associated with genitourinary anomalies.
30 Is known to be associated with a subsequent risk of malignancy.

In a child with strabismus:

31 Amblyopia is a recognized complication.
32 The diagnosis cannot be made until after 2 years of age.
33 Refractive error is an associated feature.
34 Treatment consists of patching up the good eye.
35 The diagnosis can be made if the light reflex on each cornea is asymmetrical.

A 5-week-old jaundiced infant presents with a history of passing pale stools and dark urine. The differential diagnosis includes:

36 Breast milk jaundice.
37 Neonatal hepatitis syndrome.
38 β-thalassaemia major.
39 Congenital hypothyroidism.
40 α-l-antitrypsin deficiency.

In childhood asthma:

41 An attack can be induced by exercise.
42 The disease progresses to adulthood in the majority of cases.
43 The use of salbutamol is known to be effective mainly in children over 15 months old.
44 Almost all had symptoms by 5 years of age.
45 Night cough is a recognized early presenting feature.

In an infant with seborrhoeic dermatitis:

46 The nails are typically affected.
47 The scalp is involved.
48 Pruritus is a characteristic feature.
49 Scaling is a recognized feature.
50 A family history of atopy is present in the majority of cases.

Answers

26 **False** — descent is unusual after 1 year of age. Because of
    potential irreversible changes in the germinal
    epithelium after 2 or 3 years, orchidopexy should be
    done earlier.
27 **False** — see previous answer.
28 **False.**
29 **True.**
30 **True.**

31 **True.**
32 **False.**
33 **True.**
34 **True.**
35 **True.**

36 **False** — the passage of acholic stools and dark urine suggests
    an obstructive jaundice, i.e. conjugated
    hyperbilirubinaemia. Breast-milk jaundice contains
    mainly unconjugated bilirubin.
37 **True.**
38 **False.**
39 **False** — it causes unconjugated hyperbilirubinaemia.
40 **True.**

41 **True.**
42 **False** — about 5% of asthmatic children continue to have the
    disease in adulthood.
43 **True.**
44 **True** — unfortunately not all these children are recognized as
    asthma sufferers.
45 **True.**

46 **False** — the nails are spared.
47 **True.**
48 **False** — pruritus is a feature of atopic eczema.
49 **True.**
50 **False** — there is no proved association with atopy.

Questions

Congenital adrenal hyperplasia:

51 Is a sex-linked inherited inborn error of metabolism.
52 Is a known cause of sudden infant death.
53 Is associated with cardiac arrhythmias.
54 Is characterized by low serum sodium and potassium values.
55 Presents as weight loss and vomiting during the early neonatal period.

Anencephaly:

56 Is associated with an abnormal chromosome 5.
57 Is associated with spina bifida.
58 Is associated with adrenocortical hypoplasia.
59 Is associated with hydramnios.
60 Is associated with a raised maternal plasma alphafetoprotein.

Antenatal diagnosis is available for the following conditions:

61 Thalassaemia major.
62 Neurofibromatosis.
63 Tay–Sachs disease.
64 Galactosaemia.
65 α-l-antitrypsin deficiency.

Herpes simplex infection:

66 Spares the palate in gingivostomatitis in young children.
67 Responds to local steroid treatment when confined to the skin.
68 Remains latent in the body for life.
69 Is usually caused by different strains of the organism in neonates and older children.
70 Is an indication for termination of pregnancy if a mother has active genital herpes.

In neonatal conjunctivitis:

71 Chlamydia trachomatis is a recognized cause.
72 The treatment should include a mydriatric agent.
73 There is an association with congenital rubella.
74 The pupil is characteristically small.
75 *N. gonorrhoea* infection is associated with a purulent discharge developing within the first 24 hours of life.

Answers

51 False — it is an autosomal recessive condition.
52 True.
53 True — this is related to hyperkalaemia.
54 False — serum sodium is low but potassium is raised.
55 True.

56 False — the cause is unknown. Genetic and/or environmental factors are probably involved. Excess vitamin A can produce a similar condition in rat embryos.
57 True.
58 True.
59 True.
60 True — as in open spina bifida, maternal plasma alphafetoprotein is raised.

61 True — DNA probes are available.
62 False.
63 True — this is possible at 12–16 weeks' gestation by measuring the lysosomal enzyme content (hexosaminidase) of cultured amniotic fluid cells.
64 True.
65 True — this is done by using DNA probe analysis, only at a research level at present.

66 False — it affects the mucous membranes of the mouth.
67 False — steroid is contraindicated. There is no effective topical medication although acyclovir is reported to relieve pain.
68 True — this is a general characteristic of herpes viruses.
69 True — HSV-2 infection causes genital herpes and hence is more common in neonates. HSV-1 is responsible mainly for non-genital infections and affects mainly older children and adults.
70 False — the baby should be delivered by caesarean section if the mother has active genital herpes infections, because of risk of encephalitis.

71 True.
72 False — antibiotic eye drops/ointment are the treatment of choice.
73 False.
74 False.
75 True.

Questions

Recognized features of infantile scurvy include:

76 Bone tenderness.
77 Symmetrical subperiosteal haemorrhage.
78 Bleeding gums.
79 Night-blindness.
80 Perifollicular skin bleeding.

In chickenpox infection:

81 The infectious period begins before the skin eruption appears.
82 There are characteristically more spots peripherally than centrally.
83 A life-long immunity follows an infection.
84 Vesicles on both the hard and soft palates are typical findings.
85 There is a cross-immunity to herpes simplex type II infections.

In cystic fibrosis:

86 The gene frequency is about 1 : 20 of the British population.
87 About 15% of children have a normal sweat test.
88 Sexual development is unaffected.
89 Regular daily physiotherapy is indicated even in asymptomatic children.
90 Splenomegaly due to portal hypertension is a recognized feature.

In breast-milk jaundice:

91 The infant's stools are typically clay coloured.
92 The reticulocyte count is raised.
93 The serum bilirubin is mainly unconjugated.
94 The affected infant typically fails to thrive.
95 There is an increased incidence of high-tone deafness in affected children.

Classical phenylketonuria:

96 Is inherited as an autosomal dominant with variable penetrance.
97 Demands treatment with a diet from which phenylalanine has been totally excluded.
98 Is routinely screened for on all children towards the end of the first week of life.
99 Is a recognized cause of liver damage in untreated patients.
100 Is associated with deficiency of phenylalanine hydroxylase.

Answers

76 **True** — bone tenderness is typically over the legs and may cause pseudoparalysis.
77 **True** — this is evident on X-ray during the healing stage.
78 **False** — bleeding gums are characteristic of scurvy in patients with poor dental hygiene and gingivitis.
79 **False** — this is due to vitamin A deficiency.
80 **True** — petechial haemorrhage may occur in the skin and mucous membranes.

81 **True** — the infectious stage is 1–2 days before the appearance of the rash until all the vesicles have dried up.
82 **False** — the rash is more profuse on the trunk.
83 **True.**
84 **True.**
85 **False.**

86 **True** — about 4–5% of the Caucasian population are carriers of the gene.
87 **False** — the sweat test is almost always abnormal.
88 **False** — sexual development is often delayed but only by a couple of years.
89 **True** — *Staphylococcus aureus* infection is common initially and pseudomonas infection affects the lungs later.
90 **True** — portal hypertension, oesophageal varices and hypersplenism due to biliary cirrhosis are recognized complications.

91 **False** — clay-coloured or acholic stools are indicative of an obstructive jaundice which demands immediate investigation.
92 **False** — there is no haemolysis and the reticulocyte count is normal.
93 **True.**
94 **False** — affected babies are usually well and thriving.
95 **False** — there is no evidence for this. High-tone deafness is a recognized complication in infants with kernicterus or severe hyperbilirubinaemia, but this has never been reported in breast milk jaundice.

96 **False** — phenylketonuria is an autosomal recessive inborn error of metabolism.
97 **False** — a low-phenylalanine diet is required.
98 **True** — it is called the Guthrie test which is done on capillary blood blotted onto filter paper.
99 **False** — the liver is not involved; the brain is the only significant target organ.
100 **True.**

Questions

SECTION C

Sudden infant death syndrome (SIDS):

1 Has a peak incidence in the first 2–3 months of life.
2 Occurs at night in the majority of cases.
3 Occurs less frequently in breast-fed babies.
4 Is more likely to occur in subsequent children, following an initial infant death in a family.
5 Is inherited in a complex polygenic fashion.

In classic haemophilia:

6 The disease is transmitted from an asymptomatic mother to her sons only.
7 A positive family history is obtained in less than 50% of cases.
8 The severity of the disease is not dependent on the plasma factor VIII level.
9 The hallmark of which the disease presents is haemarthrosis.
10 The partial thromboplastin time is prolonged.

Pityriasis rosea:

11 Is also called the 'Fifth disease'.
12 Is characterized by a herald patch.
13 Is characterized by a livid erythematous appearance on the cheeks ('slapped cheek') of a child.
14 Is itchy.
15 Is associated with post-inflammatory hypopigmentation.

Rubella vaccine:

16 Is contraindicated in patients with egg allergy.
17 When given to an individual will not transmit the virus to other close contacts.
18 Should be given to pregnant women who are rubella contacts.
19 Is known to cause lymphadenopathy following immunization.
20 Is recognized to cause arthralgia especially in girls.

Portwine naevus:

21 Is typically present at birth.
22 Can be treated effectively with cryotherapy.
23 Undergoes spontaneous involution in the majority of cases.
24 Is known to be associated with seizures.
25 Is known to be associated with thrombocytopenia.

Answers

1 **True** — rare before 2 weeks and after 6 months of age.
2 **True** — death usually occurs between midnight and 9 a.m.
3 **False** — breast feeding does not protect.
4 **True** — there is 5–10 times the usual risk.
5 **False** — there is no evidence for mendelian inheritance. Prenatal and postnatal (environmental) factors are more important.

6 **True** — it is a X-linked recessive inherited disorder.
7 **False** — some 80% of cases have a positive family history.
8 **False** — the severity is related to the plasma factor VIII concentration. Severe cases have 1–2% of the normal, mild cases have 6–30%.
9 **True** — knees, elbows and ankle joints are commonly involved.
10 **True** — the prothrombin and bleeding times are normal.

11 **False** — Fifth disease is erythema infectiosum which is caused by human parvovirus B19.
12 **True** — a round or oval patch may occur anywhere on the body. Fine adherent scales are present on the patch.
13 **False** — this is typical of erythema infectiosum.
14 **True.**
15 **True** — hypo or hyperpigmentation may occur especially in dark skinned patients, but these changes normally disappear after a few weeks.

16 **False** — current vaccine is a live attenuated virus vaccine prepared in human diploid cells.
17 **True** — there is no evidence that a vaccinated person can communicate the virus to others.
18 **False** — it should not be given to pregnant women because of the risk to the fetus.
19 **True** — lymphadenopathy occurs in about 20% of cases.
20 **True** — arthralgia occurs in less than 10% of cases and it occurs within 1–3 weeks of vaccination.

21 **True** — this is in contrast to strawberry naevus which are usually not present at birth but appear in the the first 2 months of life.
22 **False.**
23 **False** — it is a permanent developmental defect of the capillaries.
24 **True** — when it involves the trigeminal area of the face it may be a feature of Sturge–Weber syndrome.
25 **False** — Thrombocytopenia may be associated with large strawberry naevus.

Questions

In cleft palate:

26 There is a recognized association with other congenital malformation.
27 Surgical closure is best performed in the first 6 months of life.
28 Recurrent otitis media is a recognized complication.
29 Speech defect is known to be present even after good palatal surgery.
30 There is an increased risk of recurrence in siblings of an affected child.

A typical normal 3 year old is able to do the following:

31 Build a tower of 9 bricks.
32 Copy a cross.
33 Skip on both feet.
34 Turn pages singly.
35 Name 4 colours.

Sweat sodium is raised in the following conditions:

36 Coeliac disease.
37 Untreated adrenal insufficiency.
38 Hereditary nephrogenic diabetes insipidus.
39 Poorly controlled diabetes mellitus.
40 Hypothyroidism.

Recognized features of vitamin D deficiency rickets include:

41 Pains in the limbs.
42 A 'cracked-pot' sound on skull percussion.
43 Elevated serum phosphate.
44 Elevated serum alkaline phosphatase.
45 Delayed closure of the anterior fontanelle.

In congenital dislocation of the hip:

46 There are more girls than boys affected.
47 The Trendelenburg test is positive on the affected side.
48 Necrosis of the femoral head is a recognised complication of treatment.
49 There is a characteristic limitation of adduction.
50 There is an increased risk of recurrence in siblings of an affected child.

Answers

26 **True.**

27 **False** — most surgeons feel the palate is best repaired during the second year of life. In contrast, cleft lip is usually repaired at 1–2 months of age.

28 **True.**

29 **True** — the speech defect is due to inadequate function of the palatal and pharyngeal muscles.

30 **True** — the risk is 3% among siblings and 6.2% in offsprings.

31 **True.**

32 **False** — a 3-year-old can imitate a cross and copies one by 4 years.

33 **False** — skips on both feet at 5 years but is able to stand on one foot for seconds only.

34 **True** — able to do this by 2–2½ years.

35 **True.**

36 **False.**

37 **True.**

38 **True.**

39 **False.**

40 **True** — other causes of raised sweat electrolytes include ectodermal dysplasia, mucopolysaccharidoses, fucidosis and malnutrition.

41 **True.**

42 **False** — this is a sign for probable raised intracranial pressure. Craniotabes ('ping-pong' sensation) is a feature in vitamin D deficiency rickets.

43 **False** — this is low because the low calcium leads to increased parathormone secretion which causes a decrease in the reabsorption of phosphate in the kidney.

44 **True** — this is due to increased osteoblastic activity.

45 **True.**

46 **True** — girls are affected about four times more frequently.

47 **True** — when a child with normal hips stands on one leg, the pelvis is stabilized or levelled by the hip abductors. In a child with CDH, when weight is borne on the affected side, the pelvis drops on the opposite side because of weak hip abductors — 'positive Trendelenburg test'.

48 **True.**

49 **False** — there is limited *abduction* on the affected side caused by shortened and contracted hip adductor muscles.

50 **True** — the risk is about 4%.

Questions

Recognized features of neonatal meningitis include:

51 A bulging fontanelle.
52 Jaundice.
53 Tachypnoea.
54 Hypothermia.
55 Apnoea.

In Wilms' tumour:

56 There is a recognized association with genitourinary anomalies.
57 Metastases are to the lungs in the majority of cases.
58 Hypertension is a feature.
59 It typically presents as an abdominal mass which crosses the midline.
60 Urinary catecholamine levels are characteristically raised.

Perthes' disease:

61 Is known to affect the shoulders.
62 Is bilateral in the majority of cases.
63 Is known to present with a painless limp.
64 Affects boys in the majority of cases.
65 Typically affects preschool children.

In whooping cough:

66 The lymphocyte count is high in the peripheral blood.
67 Apnoea is a recognized feature in young infants.
68 The treatment with erythromycin will shorten the course of the disease.
69 Atelectasis is a recognized complication.
70 Subconjunctival haemorrhage is a known feature.

The following statements are true of a normal 12-month-old infant:

71 The parachute reflex is absent.
72 The asymmetrical tonic neck reflex is present.
73 The Landau reflex can be difficult to elicit.
74 The dolls' eyes response is present.
75 The Babinski reflex is present.

Answers

51 **True.**
52 **True.**
53 **True** — 70% of infants present with respiratory distress.
54 **True** — the affected infant may also be pyrexial.
55 **True.**

56 **True** — there is an association with congenital anomalies in some 13% of patients with Wilm's tumour. Genitourinary, hemihypertrophy and sporadic aniridia are common associated anomalies.
57 **True** — 80% of metastases are to the lungs. Other sites are the liver, bone and CNS.
58 **True** — this occurs in 30–60% of cases.
59 **False** — the abdominal mass seldom crosses the midline.
60 **True** — this is also raised in other abdominal tumours. There is no prognostic significance.

61 **False** — Perthes' disease is a form of osteochondritis which affects the head of the femur.
62 **False** — it is usually unilateral (over 80%).
63 **True.**
64 **True** — 80% of affected children are boys.
65 **False** — it usually affects children between 5 and 10 years old.

66 **True.**
67 **True.**
68 **False** — erythromycin may render a person non-infectious but has no effect on the course of the disease.
69 **True.**
70 **True.**

71 **True** — this reflex appears at 6–9 months and persists throughout life.
72 **False** — the asymmetrical tonic neck reflexes disappear after 6–7 months. It persists or may increase in infants with cerebral palsy.
73 **True** — this reflex is elicited by holding the infant in ventral suspension and when the head is depressed, the hip, knees and elbows flex. This is present from 1 year. Absent in cases of motor weakness, cerebral palsy and mental deficiency.
74 **False** — persistence of this response beyond the first few days of life is abnormal.
75 **True** — this response consists of flexion or extension of the big toe and movement (fanning) of the other toes when the lateral part of the sole is stimulated. It is present throughout life.

Questions

In diabetes mellitus:

76 Dietary management alone is sufficient in teenage patients.
77 A better control can only be achieved if the patient attends a special school.
78 HbA1$_c$ is a useful marker of acute diabetic control.
79 Neuropathy occurs after 5 years of poor diabetic control.
80 There is an association with histocompatibility antigen, HLA-B8.

In the cover test:

81 A true squint and pseudosquint can be differentiated.
82 If as one eye is covered and there is no movement of its fellow eye, then it implies that there is bifoveal fixation.
83 If as one eye is covered and its fellow eye moved temporally, then it implies that there was a manifest convergent squint.
84 A latent squint is detected only by watching the covered eye as the cover is removed.
85 The near fixation target should ideally be provided only at one metre.

A child on a gluten-free diet should not eat:

86 Smarties.
87 Maize.
88 Soya milks.
89 Cornflakes.
90 Bran.

Recognized features of minimal change nephrotic syndrome include:

91 A raised serum cholesterol level.
92 Haematuria is present in a minority of cases.
93 Response to steroid treatment in the majority of cases.
94 A raised serum sodium level.
95 Hypertension.

The incubation periods of the following infections are frequently more than 14 days:

96 Chickenpox.
97 *Salmonella typhimurium.*
98 Measles.
99 Mumps.
100 Hepatitis A.

Answers

76   **False** — insulin is always required. However, in a minority of cases during the 'honeymoon' period, diabetic control may be temporarily controlled without insulin injections.

77   **False.**

78   **False** — glycosylated haemoglobin is a marker of long-term control. It reflects the preceding 6–8 weeks blood glucose control.

79   **False.**

80   **True** — other associated HLA systems include HLA-BW15, DW3 and DW5.

81   **True.**

82   **False** — there is bifoveal fixation only if the test is repeated on the other eye and there is no movement.

83   **True.**

84   **True.**

85   **False** — fixative targets could be at 1/3 of a metre, 6 m and 20 m.

86   **True.**

87   **False.**

88   **False.**

89   **False.**

90   **True.**

91   **True.**

92   **True.**

93   **True.**

94   **False** — serum sodium is often decreased.

95   **False** — blood pressure is normal or low.

96   **True** — incubation period varies between 11 and 21 days but usually around 14–17 days.

97   **False** — incubation period is around 8–48 hours.

98   **False** — incubation period is around 10–12 days.

99   **True** — incubation period is 14–24 days.

100 **True** — incubation period is around 4–6 weeks.